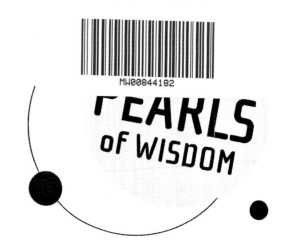

Podiatric Medicine and Surgery Part II
NATIONAL BOARD REVIEW

Second Edition

Donald Kushner, D.P.M.

McGraw-Hill
Medical Publishing Division

New York Chicago San Francisco Lisbon London
Madrid Mexico City Milan New Delhi
San Juan Seoul Singapore
Sydney Toronto

The *McGraw-Hill* Companies

Podiatric Medicine and Surgery Part II National Board Review, Second Edition

Copyright © 2006 by The McGraw-Hill Companies, Inc. All rights reserved. Printed in the United States of America. Except as permitted under the United States Copyright Act of 1976, no part of this publication may be reproduced or distributed in any form or by any means, or stored in a data base or retrieval system, without the prior written permission of the publisher.

2 3 4 5 6 7 8 9 10 DIG/DIG 09

ISBN 0-07-146448-4

Notice

Medicine is an ever-changing science. As new research and clinical experience broaden our knowledge, changes in treatment and drug therapy are required. The authors and the publisher of this work have checked with sources believed to be reliable in their efforts to provide information that is complete and generally in accord with the standards accepted at the time of publication. However, in view of the possibility of human error or changes in medical sciences, neither the authors nor the publisher nor any other party who has been involved in the preparation or publication of this work warrants that the information contained herein is in every respect accurate or complete, and they disclaim all responsibility for any errors or omissions or for the results obtained from use of the information contained in this work. Readers are encouraged to confirm the information contained herein with other sources. For example and in particular, readers are advised to check the product information sheet included in the package of each drug they plan to administer to be certain that the information contained in this work is accurate and that changes have not been made in the recommended dose or in the contraindications for administration. This recommendation is of particular importance in connection with new or infrequently used drugs.

The editors were Catherine A. Johnson and Marsha Loeb.
The production supervisor was Phil Galea.
The cover designer was Handel Low.
Von Hoffmann Graphics was printer and binder.

This book is printed on acid-free paper.

Cataloging-in-Publication data for this title is on file at the Library of Congress.

FIRST EDITION CONTRIBUTORS

Myron A. Bodman, D.P.M.
Dept. of Podiatric Medicine
Ohio College of Podiatric Medicine
Cleveland, Ohio

Georgeanne Botek, D.P.M.
Section of Podiatric Medicine
Department of Orthopaedic Surgery
Cleveland Clinic Foundation
Cleveland, Ohio

Donald E. Buddecke, D.P.M.
Broadlawns Medical Center
Des Moines, Iowa

Bryan D Caldwell, D.P.M., MS
Associate Professor, Dept. of Podiatric Medicine
Ohio College of Podiatric Medicine
Cleveland, Ohio

R.D. Lee Evans, D.P.M.
Assistant Professor of Podiatric Medicine
Shane Wortman & John Strong
College of Podiatric Medicine & Surgery
University of Osteopathic Medicine and Health
Sciences
Des Moines, Iowa

Steven L. Friedman, D.P.M.
Associate Professor
Ohio College of Podiatric Medicine
Cleveland, Ohio

John M. Giurini, D.P.M.
Beth Israel Deaconess Medical Center
Boston, Massachusetts

David W. Jenkins, D.P.M., F.A.C.F.A.S.
Associate Professor of Podiatric Medicine
College of Podiatric Medicine and Surgery
University of Osteopathic Medicine and Health
Sciences
Des Moines, Iowa

Jill Kawalec, Ph.D.
Director of Research
Ohio College of Podiatric Medicine
Cleveland, Ohio

Donald Kushner, D.P.M.
Professor and Chairman
Dept. of Podiatric Medicine
Ohio College of Podiatric Medicine
Cleveland, Ohio

Lawrence Lembach, D.P.M.
Associate Professor
Dept. of Orthopedics/Biomechanics
Ohio College of Podiatric Medicine
Cleveland, Ohio

Steven Levitz, D.P.M.
Professor
New York College of Podiatric Medicine
New York, New York

James Lichniak, D.P.M.
Associate Professor and Chairman
Dept. of Orthopedics/Biomechanics
Ohio College of Podiatric Medicine
Cleveland, Ohio

Vincent J. Mandracchia, D.P.M., MS
Director of Residency Training
Broadlawns Medical Center
Des Moines, Iowa
Clinical Professor of Podiatric Medicine
College of Podiatric Medicine and Surgery

University of Osteopathic Medicine and Health
Sciences
Des Moines, Iowa

Ewald R. Mendeszoon, D.P.M.
Beth Israel Deaconess Medical Center
Boston, Massachusetts

Travis A. Motley
College of Podiatric Medicine and Surgery
University of Osteopathic Medicine and Health
Sciences
Des Moines, Iowa

Brian J. Novack, D.P.M.
Dept. of Podiatric Surgery
Ohio College of Podiatric Medicine
Cleveland, Ohio

Kenneth W. Oglesby, D.P.M.
Beth Israel Deaconess Medical Center
Boston, Massachusetts

Lawrence Osher, D.P.M.
Professor
Dept. Of Podiatric Medicine
Ohio College of Podiatric Medicine
Cleveland, Ohio

Alpa Patel, D.P.M.
Assistant Professor
Dept. of Podiatric Medicine
Ohio College of Podiatric Medicine
Cleveland, Ohio

Hav T. Pham, D.P.M.
Beth Israel Deaconess Medical Center
Boston, Massachusetts

Jeffrey M. Robbins, D.P.M.
Director Podiatric Services
VHA Headquarters
Stokes Cleveland Veterans Affairs Medical Center
Cleveland, Ohio

Edweana Robinson, M.D.
Associate Professor
Dept. of Medicine
Ohio College of Podiatric Medicine
Cleveland, Ohio

Robert D. Rosewater, J.D.
Weston, Hurd, Fallon, Paisley, & Howley LLP
Cleveland, Ohio

Warren Rosman, J.D.
Weston, Hurd, Fallon, Paisley, & Howley LLP
Cleveland, Ohio

Ron Slate, D.P.M.
College of Podiatric Medicine and Surgery
University of Osteopathic Medicine and Health
Sciences
Des Moines, Iowa

Kevin M. Smith, D.P.M.
College of Podiatric Medicine and Surgery
University of Osteopathic Medicine and Health
Sciences
Des Moines, Iowa

Ellen Sobel, D.P.M., Ph.D.
Associate Professor
New York College of Podiatric Medicine
New York, New York

Dina Stock, D.P.M.
Assistant Professor
Department of Podiatric Medicine
Ohio College of Podiatric Medicine

Robert Weaver, D.P.M.
Assistant Professor
Dept. of Podiatric Surgery
Ohio College of Podiatric
Cleveland, Ohio

Justin Wernick, D.P.M.
Clinical Professor
New York College of Podiatric Medicine
New York, New York

INTRODUCTION

Congratulations! *Podiatric Medicine and Surgery Part II National Board Review: Pearls of Wisdom* will help you pass the national boards and improve your board scores. This book's unique format differs from all other review and test preparation texts. Let us begin, then, with a few words on purpose, format, and use.

The primary intent of this book is to serve as a rapid review of podiatric principles and serve as a study aid to improve performance on podiatric written and practical examinations. With this goal in mind, the text is written in rapid-fire, question/answer format. The student receives immediate gratification with a correct answer. Questions themselves often contain a "pearl" reinforced in association with the question/answer.

Additional hooks are often attached to the answer in various forms, including mnemonics, evoked visual imagery, repetition and humor. Additional information not requested in the question may be included in the answer. The same information is often sought in several different questions. Emphasis has been placed on evoking both trivia and key facts that are easily overlooked, are quickly forgotten, and yet somehow always seem to appear on podiatric exams.

Many questions have answers without explanations. This is done to enhance ease of reading and rate of learning. Explanations often occur in a later question/answer. It may happen that upon reading an answer the reader may think - "Hmm, why is that?" or, "Are you sure?" If this happens to you, GO CHECK! Truly assimilating these disparate facts into a framework of knowledge absolutely requires further reading in the surrounding concepts. Information learned, as a response to seeking an answer to a particular question is much better retained than that passively read. Take advantage of this. Use this book with your podiatric text handy and open, or, if you are reviewing on train, plane, or camelback, mark questions for further investigation.

Podiatric Medicine and Surgery Part II National Board Review: Pearls of Wisdom risks accuracy by aggressively pruning complex concepts down to the simplest kernel. The dynamic knowledge base and clinical practice of medicine is not like that! This text is designed to maximize your score on a test. Refer to your mentors for direction on current practice.

Podiatric Medicine and Surgery Part II National Board Review: Pearls of Wisdom is designed to be used, not just read. It is an interactive text. Use a 3x5 card and cover the answers; attempt all questions. A study method we strongly recommend is oral, group study, preferably over an extended meal or pitchers. The mechanics of this method are simple and no one ever appears stupid. One person holds the book, with answers covered, and reads the question. Each person, including the reader, says "Check!" when he or she has an answer in mind. After everyone has "checked" in, someone states his or her answer. If this answer is correct, on to the next one. If not, another person states his or her answer, or the answer can be read. Usually, the person who "checks" in first gets the first shot at stating the answer. If this person is being a smarty-pants answer-hog, then others can take turns. Try it—it's almost fun!

Podiatric Medicine and Surgery Part II National Board Review: Pearls of Wisdom is also designed to be re-used several times to allow, dare we use the word, memorization. I suggest putting a check mark in the hollow bullet provided when a question is missed. A hollow bullet has been arbitrarily provided. If you answer a question incorrectly again on re-uses of this book, forget this question! You will get it wrong on the exam! Another suggestion is to place a check mark when the question is answered correctly once; skip all questions with check marks thereafter. Utilize whatever scheme of using the bullets you prefer.

We welcome your comments, suggestions and criticism. Great effort has been made to verify these questions and answers. There will be answers we have provided that are at variance with the answer you would prefer. Most often this is attributable to the variance between original source (previously discussed). Please make us aware of any errata you find. We hope to make continuous improvements in future editions and would greatly appreciate any input with regard to format, organization, content, presentation, or about specific questions. Please write to Donald Kushner at dkushner@ocpm.edu. We look forward to hearing from you.

Study hard and good luck!

D.K.

TABLE OF CONTENTS

ANESTHESIA

○ **Which level of anesthesia is considered surgical anesthesia?**

Level III.

○ **There are four reflexes progressively lost in level III anesthesia. The third reflex lost in the progression is?**

Thoracic muscular.

○ **While performing an Austin bunionectomy under General anesthesia, you over hear the Anesthesiologist mention that he/she is administering Reglan. What is this for?**

Reduce gastric motility.

○ **Pediatric hypoglycemia is extremely dangerous! Pediatric patients have a very limited amount of glycogen stores, and therefore should always have what fluid running in their IV?**

D5W.

○ **What are the effects of low serum calcium on the EKG?**

With a wide QRS complex.

○ **What effect does Ketamine have on a patient?**

Amnesia only.

○ **Fentanyl is used as what?**

Narcotic analgesic.

○ **What drug has largely replaced Sodium Pentothal?**

Diprivan.

○ **What is the first symptom of malignant hyperthermia?**

Tachycardia.

○ **Describe the mechanism of breakdown for Esters & Amides.**

Esters are hydrolyzed by pseudocholinesterase in plasma; amides are metabolized in the liver.

○ **What is the treatment for convulsions?**

Valium.

❍   **Describe a Mayo block.**

Local "ring" block of the 1st metatarsophalangeal joint.

❍   **Describe MAC anesthesia.**

IV sedation with a local anesthesia block.

❍   **How does local anesthesia provide pain relief?**

Prevents sodium migration through the nerve membrane, which prevents depolarization and causes inhibition of nerve conduction.

❍   **What is the basic treatment for shock?**

Fluids, ABC's, monitor vitals.

❍   **The American Society of Anesthesiologists surgical risk classification system classifies "A healthy patient" as what class?**

Class I.

❍   **List the complications associated with tourniquet use?**

Tissue necrosis, Inflammation, Paralysis, Thrombosis, Circulatory volume overload.

❍   **A contraindication to Tourniquet use would be?**

Previous Popliteal- Dorsalis pedis bypass grafting. Sickle cell disease is potentially a contraindication as well, because the tourniquet causes low oxygen tension which could cause cells to sickle.

❍   **List the potential complications of Endotracheal Intubation?**

Sore throat, Tracheal edema, Croup, laceration, pneumothorax.

❍   **When positioning a patient in the supine position during general anesthesia, the most common complication is?**

Ulnar nerve neuropathy.

❍   **When positioning a patient in the prone position during general anesthesia, the most common complication is?**

Pressure on the orbit as well as the dorsum of the foot.

❍   **During Spinal anesthesia, the space in the lumbar area of the spine into which the anesthetic is placed is the?**

Subarachnoid space, deep to the dura.

❍   **Complications of spinal anesthesia include?**

Headache, Hypotension, Cauda equina syndrome, and infection.

○ **What is the most common cause of temperature elevation intraoperatively?**

Malignant hyperthermia.

○ **What medication is used to treat Malignant Hyperthermia?**

Dantrolene IV.

○ **What type of allergic reaction is Anaphylaxis?**

A type I antibody mediated hypersensitivity reaction, seen immediately.

○ **What are early signs of Anaphylaxis?**

Flush, difficulty in breathing, wheezing, stridor, laryngeal edema.

○ **What is the treatment for Anaphylaxis?**

Epinephrine 0.3-0.5 ml sub Q of a 1:1,000 solution, along with antihistamines.

○ **Describe the mechanism of action of local anesthetics.**

Local anesthetics prevent conduction of the nerve by decreasing sodium permeability thus increasing the excitation threshold.

○ **What is the toxic dose of Lidocaine 1% plain?**

300mg (30ml).

○ **What is the toxic dose of Lidocaine 1% with Epinephrine?**

500mg (50ml).

○ **What is toxic dose of Bupivacaine 0.25% plain?**

175mg (70ml).

○ **What is the toxic dose of Bupivacaine 0.25% with Epinephrine?**

225mg (90ml).

○ **List four common Amide based local anesthetics.**

Lidocaine, Bupivacaine, Mepivacaine, and Etidocaine.

○ **List four common ester based local anesthetics.**

Procaine, Tetracaine, Chloroprocaine, and hexylcaine.

○ **When performing tendon transfer type procedures list the type of potential anesthesia that may be used.**

General, Spinal, and Epidural (because each of these modalities will temporarily eliminate lower extremity muscular activity).

O   **What type of local block is most widely accepted when performing HAV surgery in a healthy patient?**

MAC with local Mayo block.

O   **What nerve lies within the first intermetatarsal space?**

Deep peroneal.

O   **What nerve lies anterior to the medial malleolus?**

Saphenous.

O   **Cervical spine radiographs should be obtained on a patient with a history of ?**

Rheumatoid arthritis.

O   **When using a high thigh tourniquet, which types of anesthesia would be unwise?**

MAC, and local types because the high thigh tourniquet causes too much discomfort and generally requires a general anesthetic.

O   **The recommended pressure for a high thigh tourniquet is?**

200 mm Hg over systolic pressure due to the large soft tissue mass in the thigh.

O   **During which stage of anesthesia would it be appropriate to elevate an extremity tourniquet?**

Stage II.

O   **When comparing a spinal block to a epidural block which will allow greater control?**

Epidural block.

O   **When a patient has just completed general anesthesia and is violently shaking as if cold, which medication will relieve these symptoms?**

Demerol.

O   **On the morning of surgery a patient with non-insulin dependent diabetes, hypothyroidism, and hypertension should be told to take all of their medication except?**

They should not take their oral hypoglycemic because they have been NPO and could become severely hypoglycemic and go into insulin shock.

O   **True or false - The toxic dose of local anesthetics is increased with the addition of epinephrine to the anesthetic.**

True. Epinephrine slows the absorption of the anesthetic and therefore allows more to be used.

O   **Anesthesia is defined as?**

Loss of sensation with or without the loss of consciousness.

○ **Factors that affect the concentration of a drug at a site of action, as a function of time is referred to as?**

Pharmacokinetics.

○ **Succinylcholine is primarily used to achieve?**

Muscle relaxation through depolarization.

○ **Succinylcholine can cause what adverse reactions?**

Fasciculations as well as hyperkalemia.

○ **List a potential adverse reaction caused by the drug Toradol?**

It can cause a peptic ulcer.

○ **Do ester type anesthetics have a higher or lower allergic potential than Amides?**

Higher.

○ **The protein-binding characteristic of a drug will affect what?**

Duration of action.

○ **Is eating within 6 hours prior to a general anesthetic a cause to cancel the surgery?**

Yes, due to the risk of regurgitation and aspiration.

○ **During a local field block what sensation is lost first?**

Pain and temperature first, second is touch and motor.

○ **A local field block injected into an infected area is less active because of what action?**

The acidic area of the infection converts the anesthetic chemically thus decreasing penetration into the cell membrane.

○ **When performing an ankle block which nerves are blocked?**

Saphenous, Posterior Tibial, Sural, Superficial Peroneal, and Deep Peroneal.

○ **When performing various types of anesthesia on pediatric patients what is the common concern during anesthesia?**

Hypothermia (temperature fluctuations).

○ **What is the drug of choice to increase the threshold of convulsions during the intraoperative period?**

Valium.

○ **What are the initial steps to perform once it is determined the patient is having a syncope reaction?**

Oxygen, Trendelenburg positioning, monitor vitals.

❍ **Wydases works by what action?**

Permitting a more rapid spread of solution into the area.

❍ **When using Halothane, what vasoconstrictive drug is contraindicated?**

Epinephrine.

❍ **What are the adverse effects of narcotics?**

Respiratory depression, emesis, and dependence.

❍ **Which inhalation agent is nonflammable?**

Halothane.

❍ **Esters are hydrolyzed in the _____?**

Plasma (higher allergic potential!).

❍ **Amides are metabolized in the _____?**

Liver.

❍ **What type of anesthesia causes the least interference with preexisting diseases?**

Regional nerve block.

❍ **During surgery if a patient becomes hyperkalemic what may you observe?**

Muscle weakness, cardiac conduction (EKG) changes.

❍ **Which has a greater duration of action Lidocaine or Marcaine?**

Marcaine.

❍ **What are the various etiologies of syncope?**

Syncope may be due to many etiologies including vasovagal, postural hypotension, chronic orthostatic hypotension, cardiac, carotid sinus, secondary to cerebrovascular disease, etc.

ARTHROSCOPY

○ **Portals should be separated as widely as possible, consistent with the anatomy, to avoid this?**

Skin necrosis due to the portals placed too close to each other.

○ **If an instrument fails or breaks within the joint, what should be done immediately?**

Outflow of saline should be shut down while the inflow is left open to keep the joint distended for retrieval of the broken piece.

○ **What anatomical structures are considered when making an anterolateral portal?**

Between the extensor digitorum longus and the superficial peroneal nerve.

○ **When is the transmalleolar approach for lesions of the talus contraindicated?**

In children with open epiphyses.

○ **What anatomical structures should be considered when making an anteromedial portal?**

Between the saphenous vein and the tibialis anterior tendon.

○ **What is the most common size and angulation of an arthroscope used in an ankle?**

2.7 mm and 30 degrees or 0 degrees of angulation.

○ **What is the minimum distance an accessory portal should be placed between the two working portals?**

At least 1 cm apart to avoid skin necrosis.

○ **How would one confirm that the loose body seen on x-ray is intra-articular instead of intra-capsular or extra-articular?**

Perform an arthrogram, perhaps in combination with a CT or MRI.

○ **In anterior soft tissue impingement of the ankle, pathology is generally limited to what?**

The syndesmosis and the lateral gutter.

○ **When using the posterolateral approach, one should avoid what anatomical structures?**

Subcutaneous sural nerve or the short saphenous vein. Also avoid entering the STJ.

○ **Transmalleolar portals are more often required on which side of the ankle joint and why?**

On the medial side because lateral dome lesions are more anterior than on the medial side, and because the lateral malleolus is further posterior than the medial malleolus.

❍   **What are three basic joint surveying techniques in ankle arthroscopy?**

Scanning, pistoning, and rotating.

❍   **Prior to beginning arthroscopy, which portal is developed first?**

The medial portal is developed first and the scope is placed in to survey the joint prior to lateral portal development.

❍   **What are the contraindications for manual distraction and/or gravity distraction?**

Tight ankles, pathology not easily accessible, and prolonged procedures.

❍   **What are the contraindications to the use of non-invasive distraction?**

Impaired circulatory status, diabetes, generalized medical conditions, ankle edema, or fragile skin.

❍   **What are the contraindications to the use of skeletal distraction?**

Local or generalized infections, osteopenia, open epiphysis, and lax ligaments.

❍   **What are some of the indications for the use of single heavy pin distraction (3/16 inch)?**

Large bone structure in males, long cases or difficult pathology, very tight ankles, ankle arthrodesis, etc.

❍   **What are some advantages of double pin (7/64 inch) distraction?**

Better control, less stress riser than 3/16 inch, less chance of pin tract infection.

❍   **What are the recommended parameters of force and duration for non-invasive distraction?**

20-25 lbs of force for about 30-45 minutes.

❍   **What are the parameters for proximal pin placement in skeletal distraction?**

3/16 or 7/64 inserted 2 inches; 2 ¼ up to 4 inches above ankle joint usually from the lateral side.

❍   **What are the three insertion sites for distal pin placement in skeletal distraction?**

Two in the calcaneus and one in the talus.

❍   **How is the distal pin inserted in the calcaneus?**

It is inserted at a 20-25 degree downward slope so that when distraction occurs the pin will become parallel with the proximal pin.

❍   **What size of pin is used in light double distraction mode?**

7/64¼smooth pins.

❍   **What size of pin is used in heavy single or double distraction?**

3/16¼threaded pin.

❍ **When a 3/16½ invasive distraction is used, how long post-operatively should the patient avoid athletic activity or heavy work?**

With heavy distraction, the patient should avoid athletic activity or heavy work for 8-10 weeks to decrease the risk of fracture.

❍ **When 7/64½ invasive distraction is used, when can the patient return to activity?**

Four to six weeks.

❍ **What type of specific synovitis occurs in three stages?**

Chronic synovial chondromatosis.

❍ **Which disease entity is characterized by synovitis with advanced papillary formation and hemosiderin cells present?**

Pigmented villonodular synovitis.

❍ **Osteochondral lesions of the talar dome are commonly found where?**

Commonly found at the anterior lateral aspect or the posterior medial aspect of the dome.

❍ **What is the mechanism of injury in a medial talar dome osteochondral lesion?**

Inversion of the foot with ankle plantarflexed.

❍ **What is the mechanism of injury in a lateral talar dome osteochondral lesion?**

Inversion of the foot with the ankle dorsiflexed and tibia internally rotated on the talus.

❍ **What is used in drilling an osteochondral lesion of the talar dome?**

0.062 Kirschner wire.

❍ **How should a bone graft be placed in the articular cartilage of the talar dome?**

The graft should be placed 1-2 mm below the level of the articular cartilage.

❍ **What is one method that has been proven helpful in viewing chondral lesions of the ankle joint?**

The use of methylene blue dye injected into the joint and then washed out with irrigant saline.

❍ **What technique is used in arthroscopic ankle arthrodesis?**

Arthroscopic transmalleolar cross-screw fusion.

❍ **What are some advantages of the arthroscopic approach to ankle fusion over the open method?**

Less surgical morbidity and improved cosmesis.

❍ **What is a disadvantage of the arthroscopic approach to ankle fusion?**

Severe varus/valgus malalignment is difficult to correct arthroscopically.

○   **What is a contraindication to doing arthroscopic ankle fusion?**

A varus/valgus malalignment greater than 15 degrees.

○   **What type and size of screw is used in arthroscopic ankle fusion to fuse the ankle?**

Cannulated 6.5 mm cancellous screw system.

○   **What are considered abnormal values in the anterior drawer stress test?**

Between 5-10 mm of anterior displacement of the talus from the distal tibia are considered abnormal, and over 10 mm of displacement are considered grossly abnormal. In comparison with the unaffected extremity, the injured ankle should have an anterior drawer test result of 3 mm or more to be considered significant.

○   **Name the arthroscopic technique that involves insertion of another object such as a probe beside a target structure into the field of view of the arthroscope in order for the physician to better conceptualize the relative positions of these objects to one another or adjacent structures.**

Triangulation.

○   **According to R.W. Jackson (1982), is more relief of symptoms achieved with diagnostic arthroscopy attributable to joint lavage or lyses of adhesions?**

Joint lavage 21%; lysis of adhesions 4%.

○   **What does the Berndt and Hardy classification system classify? Describe it.**

Transchondral fractures: Stage I – Compression of the articular cartilage, Stage II – An incomplete fracture, Stage III – A non-displaced complete fracture, Stage IV – Displaced complete fracture.

○   **Which side of the anterior half of the talar dome usually produces a shallow wafer-shaped fracture?**

Lateral.

○   **Which side of the posterior third of the talar dome is subject to deep, cup-shaped lesions?**

Medial.

○   **What is the procedure for sterilization of an arthroscope?**

First case – Ethylene oxide gas, Additional cases – Activated glutaraldehyde solution for 20 minutes. Arthroscopes cannot be autoclaved.

○   **What is the probable diagnosis if only 10-12 ml of saline can be injected into the ankle joint capsule of a normal size adult?**

Capsular adhesions or fibrosis.

○   **Plantarflexion of the foot increases the visualization for which group of arthroscopic portal approaches?**

Anterior.

O **Dorsiflexion of the foot increases the visualization for which group of arthroscopic portal approaches?**

Posterior.

O **Name the indications for ankle joint arthroscopy:**

Chronic ankle instability, persistent ankle joint pain, ankle fractures, ankle fusions, arthritis, (rheumatoid and osteoarthritis), adhesive capsulitis, synovitis, menoscoid bodies, chondromalacia, chondral and osteochondral defects, arterior impingement exostosis, and pre-operative planning.

O **Name and describe the three principles or maneuvers performed in arthroscopy.**

Pistoning is the movement of the arthroscope toward or away from an object. Pistoning toward an object would increase the object's apparent size while decreasing the total field of vision. Scanning or sweeping is the side to side or up and down movement of the arthroscope to get a more complete view of a joint. The idea is to go from known to unknown areas of the joint to distinguish normal from pathological structures. Rotation is the movement of the arthroscope about its axis. The field of vision is changed depending on the obliquity of the arthroscope tip. The larger the degree of tip cut, the wider the field.

O **The first person to perform an endoscopic intra-articular observation (1918) and also the first successful ankle arthroscopy?**

Takagi – University of Tokyo.

O **What instrument has a sharp point and is used to pierce soft tissue and capsule?**

Trocar.

O **What instrument has a blunt point and is used to enter a joint? Why?**

Obturator, To prevent iatrogenic cartilaginous damage.

O **Arthroscopes are available in what sizes?**

1.7 mm to 8.0 mm.

O **What is used to distend the ankle joint and maintain a clean field for the camera?**

Irrigation system of normal saline.

O **For chondromalacia, osteochondral defects, and osteoarthritis, burrs are used to abrade articular defects to what level?**

Viable bleeding bone.

O **What structure is the landmark for locating the proper site for an anteromedial portal approach for an ankle arthroscopy?**

Tibialis anterior tendon. (Must go medial to it.)

O **An anterocentral portal is always located lateral to what structure?**

EHL .

O   **What nerves are at risk of being injured with the five different portals of entry into the ankle joint?**

Anteromedial – Saphenous nerve.
Anterocentral – Deep peroneal nerve.
Anterolateral – Terminal branches of superficial peroneal nerve.
Posterior medial – Posterior tibial nerve.
Posterior lateral – Sural nerve.

O   **What is the purpose of a stopcock, on the sidearm of a cannula?**

The ingress or egress of fluids.

O   **What are the three types of light sources used in arthroscopy?**

Xenon, quartz halogen, incandescent (tungsten halogen).

O   **The three main types of motorized shower tips attach to hand engines of power arthroscopy instrumentation are the open-ended, side-cutter, and full radius. Which tip contains a normal rotating blade that prevents inadvertent damage to cartilage? Which tip is the most aggressive?**

The full radius type of tip has a round rotating blade. The open-ended tip is the most aggressive type because the end of the blade is completely exposed.

O   **Are the flutes in the sphere of an abrader more aggressive in cutting in a forward or reverse direction?**

Forward.

O   **How does the force of suction affect the aggressiveness of a shaver? An abrader?**

It increases the aggressiveness of both by aspirating more tissue into the openings at the end of the instruments.

O   **How does the speed of rotations of its blades affect a shaver? An abrader?**

The slower a shaver rotates, the more aggressively it cuts. The faster an abrader moves, the more aggressively it cuts.

O   **What two bones are the mechanical distraction system hooked into?**

Lower tibia and the calcaneus.

O   **What radiographic view is used to evaluate an anterior drawer test?**

Lateral.

O   **How many degrees of varus tilt are needed before an inversion stress test is considered abnormal?**

15 degrees when compared to the unaffected ankle.

O   **What radiographic projection is used to evaluate an inversion stress test?**

AP projection.

○   What color or appearance does synovial fluid have normally? In an inflammatory process? In the presence of gout or rheumatoid arthritis?

Normally – clear, light, pale yellow. With inflammation, turbid. With gout or rheumatoid arthritis, milky.

○   **How is the size of an arthroscope determined?**

By the diameter of the casting that contains the lens system.

○   **What determines the obliquity or direction of the field of view seen through an arthroscope?**

The tip cut of the end of the arthroscope.

○   **What are the two commonly used lens systems for arthroscopes?**

Rod lens (Hopkins) and the GRIN (Gradient Index).

○   **Abrasion arthroplasty resects necrotic islands of cartilage and/or subchondral bone to what depth? Why?**

1.0 mm (to the level of the tidemark) below the surface of subchondral bone. Because this is the area that contains the vascularity that provides nutrition to support growth of new healthy hyaline cartilage.

○   **How far above the patient must bags used for a gravity ingress system be placed?**

2-3 meters.

○   **If visualization of the ankle joint is not adequate using the anterocentral portal, which anterior portal is the best alternative? Why?**

Anteromedial because of a lack of ligamentous structures and due to the fact it has the least amount of pathology associated with it. Therefore, it is less apt to have hypertrophic synovial tissue within it.

○   **What type of portal allows for flushing and rinsing of a joint?**

Egress portal.

○   **What is the term used to describe soft tissue pathology that involves the hypertrophy of normal anatomic structures secondary to the inflammatory process?**

Impingement syndrome.

○   **Of ligaments, joint capsules, and synovial membranes, which does not have a rich supply of nerves?**

Synovial membrane.

○   **How would an acute synovitis appear differently from a chronic synovitis arthroscopically?**

Acute synovitis presents with long transparent hypertrophic villi and of uniform length, with an enlarged central vessel (injected) or a vessel that has ruptured (hemorrhagic hypertrophic synovitis). Chronic hypertrophic synovitis is neither transparent nor hemorrhagic and presents with frayed opaque villi of different lengths secondary to necrosis of their tips.

❍   **Fibers of what ligament make up the floor of the medial gutter?**

Anterior tibiotalar ligament of the deep deltoid.

❍   **The medial bend is a part of the anatomy of what bone?**

The tibia.

❍   **What is the name of the depression in the talar surface that runs from anterior to posterior near the anterocentral portion of the ankle joint?**

Sagittal groove.

❍   **The anterior tibial lip is made of what substance?**

Hyaline cartilage.

❍   **The synovial recess is made of what substance?**

Periosteum-covered subchondral bone.

❍   **What is the name of the area between the tibial tubercle, the fibula, and the lateral shoulder of the talus?**

The lateral interval.

❍   **What is the redundant joint capsule attached on top of the synovial recess of the tibia called?**

Capsular reflection.

❍   **What is the name of the arthroscopic procedure in which one resects hypertrophic synovial tissue? What cutting instrument is used to remove this tissue?**

Synovectomy; shaver or punch or suction punch.

❍   **What is the name of the arthroscopic procedure in which one debrides uneven or fibrillated cartilagenous tissue from an ankle joint?**

Chondroplasty.

❍   **Does a properly performed chondroplasty initiate cartilage repair? Why or why not?**

No, because chondroplasty only smoothes out the fibrillated or uneven portions of cartilage and does not revascularize the actual defect.

BIOMATERIALS

○ **What is the definition of a biomaterial?**

A biomaterial can be defined as a natural or synthetic material that is used to supplement or replace the functions of living tissues.

○ **List the two general types of implants, and give examples of each.**

Transient implants are those which are intended to remain in contact with the body for a temporary period of time. They then are either removed or resorbed by the body. Examples of transient implants are sutures, dressings and fixation devices. Permanent implants are those that are intended to remain in the body permanently. Examples of permanent implants include heart valves and joint replacement devices.

○ **What is biocompatibility?**

The biocompatibility of a material must consider both the host's response to a material and the physiological effect of the environment on the material.

○ **What are the two categories of biocompatibility that are essential in biomaterials?**

Biologic biocompatibility relates to the reaction of the host to the implant. The material must not cause harm to the host tissue. Mechanical biocompatibility relates to the compatibility between the properties of the material and its intended function. The material must be able to perform in a manner that is favorable to the tissue that it is enhancing or replacing.

○ **Which characteristics of a biomaterial or device can affect the host response to that material or implant?**

The shape of a material or device can adversely effect the host response. For instance, a device with sharp corners may be less compatible that a device with smoother contours. The size of a material may also affect the biological response to a material or device. For instance, a material may have excellent biocompatibility in bulk form, but may elicit a severe response in particulate form. Finally, the surface texture of a material or device may affect the host response with tissue such as bone adhering to a textured surface.

○ **What is the most commonly used test of mechanical properties of a material?**

The tensile test is the method most often used to evaluate the mechanical properties of a material. With this technique, a material is stretched at a constant rate, while the force applied to the material and the elongation of the material is measured.

○ **What are the definitions of stress and strain?**

Stress is defined as the ratio of applied force to cross-sectional area. Strain is defined as the ratio of change in length to the original length of the material specimen.

○ **What is a stress-strain curve?**

The stress-strain curve is a graph of stress versus strain. Stress is plotted on the vertical axis, or y-axis, and strain is plotted on the horizontal axis, or x-axis. The stress-strain curve depicts the change in shape (or strain) of a material for a given force (or stress).

○   **What are the two major regions on a stress-strain curve?**

The elastic region of the stress-strain curve is the initial linear (straight) portion of the curve. In this region, deformation occurs but the material returns to its original shape upon removal of the force. The plastic region of the stress-strain curve is the nonlinear portion of the curve. In this region, permanent (plastic) deformation occurs, and the material does not return to its original shape upon removal of the force.

○   **What are the three major points on a stress-strain curve?**

The yield point is the point on the stress-strain curve where the linear portion ends, and the nonlinear portion begins. It indicates the point at which elastic behavior ends, and subsequent deformation will be permanent. The ultimate tensile strength is the point of maximum stress on the stress-strain curve. It is the maximum stress that a material can withstand. The failure strength is the point of stress on the stress-strain curve where fracture occurs. It is also referred to as the fracture strength.

○   **What is the modulus of elasticity of a material?**

The modulus of elasticity is a material property related to the slope of the linear portion of the stress-strain curve. It is used to indicate the stiffness of a material. This property is often used when comparing the mechanical properties of biomaterials. If the slope of the stress-strain curve is steep, then the modulus of elasticity is high and the material is relatively stiff. In contrast, a less stiff material has a low modulus of elasticity.

○   **What is the difference between the stiffness of a material and the stiffness of a device?**

The stiffness of a material is an inherent material property, and is constant for each material. The stiffness of a device can be varied, and depends on the modulus of elasticity of the material as well as the dimensions of the device.

○   **What is the ductility of a material?**

Ductility is a measure of the degree of plastic deformation sustained at fracture. It can be expressed as either percent elongation or percent area reduction.

○   **What is the difference between a brittle material and a ductile material?**

A ductile material experiences a substantial degree of plastic deformation prior to failure. In contrast, a brittle material undergoes very little or no plastic deformation prior to failure. Brittle materials fracture before a high enough stress to produce plastic deformation is attained.

○   **What is the toughness of a material?**

Toughness is a measure of the amount of energy a material absorbs at the time of failure. It is represented by the area under the stress-strain curve, up to the point of fracture.

○   **What is the hardness of a material?**

Hardness is a measure of a material's resistance to localized plastic deformation. It relates directly to the wear of a material. The hardness of a material is determined by measuring the indentation made in a flat surface of the material by a known force.

❍ What is wear?

Wear is a process by which material is progressively lost as a result of two surfaces sliding against one another. Adhesive wear occurs when two materials in articulation with one another bond together and then dislodge as the materials continue to slide past each other. As a result, debris from one material is transferred to the surface of the other. Abrasive wear occurs when a hard material tears through another softer, more ductile material.

❍ What is fatigue failure?

Fatigue failure is a method of delayed failure resulting from fluctuating, or cyclic, stresses. It depends on the combination of the stress applied and the number of loading cycles. The greater the stress, the lower the number of cycles needed to induce failure. Fatigue failure results from crack initiation and subsequent propagation of the crack with each load cycle.

❍ What is the fatigue limit?

The fatigue limit is the stress below which fatigue failure will not occur, regardless of the number of load cycles. It varies for different materials, and not all materials have a fatigue limit. The fatigue limit is also called the endurance limit.

❍ What is viscoelasticity?

Viscoelasticity describes the viscous and elastic properties typical of polymers and biological materials. When a force is applied to a material, the initial deformation is the elastic component of viscoelasticity, and upon removal of the force, the material will retain its original shape. The viscous component of viscoelasticity is the permanent deformation that occurs. This permanent deformation is time-dependent, and increases continuously for as long as the force is applied.

❍ What is creep?

Creep is a permanent deformation that occurs over time as a result of an applied constant stress. It is a manifestation of viscoelasticity.

❍ What are the three categories of materials used as biomaterials?

The three categories of materials used as biomaterials are metals, polymers and ceramics.

❍ What are the general characteristics of metals?

Metals, in general, have a high modulus of elasticity, high mechanical strength, high yield point, and are susceptible to corrosion. Due to their mechanical properties, metals are used in applications where the device is subjected to high loads.

❍ Name the three metals most often used as biomaterials?

The three most commonly used metals are titanium alloys, cobalt-chromium alloys, and stainless steels.

❍ What is metal sensitivity?

Sensitivity is a biological reaction that may occur in response to metal implants. Also referred to as a hypersensitivity or allergic response, sensitivity results from an immune reaction to a foreign material. The primary form of sensitivity observed with metal implants is Type IV hypersensitivity. The reaction is a delayed response, and is primarily a cell-mediated process. The manifestations of metal sensitivity include contact dermatitis and a sustained inflammatory reaction that results in osteolysis.

○   **Which metal sensitivities are most common in the human population?**

Nickel sensitivity is the most common, with approximately 15% of the population exhibiting an allergic response to the metal. Stainless steels contain 13-15.5% nickel. To a lesser extent, sensitivities to chromium and cobalt also exist. The sensitivity reaction may be severe enough to necessitate removal of the device that is causing the response.

○   **What is stress shielding?**

Stress shielding is a phenomenon by which bone mass is decreased over an extended period of time as a result of the presence of a rigid device. If bone is not subjected to a significant physiological load, then the bone mass will slowly decrease. When a rigid device that has a higher stiffness than bone, such as a metal implant, is placed adjacent to bone, the applied stress is transferred to the metal. As a result, the metal effectively shields the bone from the stress, and the bone may undergo atrophy and loss of mass.

○   **What can be done to reduce stress shielding in fracture fixation?**

Less rigid, or flexible, fracture fixation devices are preferred to reduce the effects of stress shielding. Materials that have a modulus of elasticity similar to that of bone are appropriate for less rigid fracture fixation. Such materials include polymers and composites. Metals may also be used if the stiffness of the device as a whole can be reduced by varying the thickness of the fixation plate.

○   **What are the general characteristics of polymers?**

Polymers, in general, have a low modulus of elasticity, low mechanical strength, undergo time-dependent degradation and are susceptible to abrasion.

○   **Give examples of polymers that are commonly used as biomaterials.**

Examples of polymers used as biomaterials are silicone rubbers, polymethyl methacrylate (PMMA), polyethylene and absorbable polymers.

○   **What are absorbable polymers?**

Absorbable polymers are materials that degrade over time by a hydrolysis mechanism. The rate of degradation is such that, as the device loses strength, the healing tissue is able to assume the load. Eventually the polymer is solubilized or phagocytosed.

○   **What are some applications of absorbable polymers?**

Absorbable materials are used for internal fixation devices, drug delivery systems, bone fillers, wound care products, tissue scaffolds and nerve guides.

○   **List several examples of absorbable polymers.**

Absorbable materials include polyglycolic acid (PGA), polylactic acid (PLA), polydioxanone, and copolymers of PGA and PLA.

○   **What are the ideal characteristics of an absorbable fixation device?**

An absorbable fixation device should exhibit stability, with good biocompatibility, adequate mechanical strength, and a modulus of elasticity similar to that of bone. It should be non-toxic and water-soluble. Finally, it must have a predictable degradation rate.

O **What are the general characteristics of ceramics?**

Ceramics, in general, are much stronger in compression that in tension. They are brittle, and have good corrosion resistance and excellent biocompatibility.

O **List examples of ceramics that are used as biomaterials.**

Ceramics that are used as biomaterials include alumina, zirconia, carbons, hydroxyapatite, and glass ceramics.

O **List the three types of carbon that have biomedical applications.**

The three types of carbon that have biomedical applications are pyrolytic carbon, vitreous (or glassy) carbon, and vapor-deposited carbon.

O **What are the biomedical applications of pyrolytic carbon?**

Pyrolytic carbon is used for heart valves, hand and toe joints, and dental implants.

O **What are the properties of hydroxyapatite?**

Hydroxyapatite is similar in composition to the mineral component of bone. It has excellent biocompatibility and forms a direct chemical bond to hard tissues. The mechanical properties of hydroxyapatite vary widely, due to differences in manufacturing, but generally have a modulus of elasticity similar to that of bone.

O **What are the applications of hydroxyapatite?**

Hydroxyapatite can be used as porous or solid implants. It can be used as a coating on implants or as filler for gaps in bone.

O **What are glass ceramics?**

Glass ceramics consist of phosphorus, sodium, silicon and calcium components. They produce a direct bond with bone by forming a calcium-phosphate layer. The composition of glass ceramics must adhere strictly to guidelines, in order to attain bone-bonding capabilities.

O **List some applications of glass ceramics.**

Glass ceramics are used as composites, fillers for bone cement, and coatings on implants.

O **What is a composite material?**

A composite material is a combination of two or more materials, which together enhance the overall properties of the composite material. It often consists of a fiber material embedded in a matrix material. The matrix material is most often a polymer or ceramic, while the most commonly used fiber material is carbon. The main advantage of composite materials is that the properties of the composite can be tailored to the specific needs of the material.

O **What are the important considerations for orthopedic implants?**

Materials used for orthopedic implants should have a modulus of elasticity similar to bone, sufficient fatigue strength, high wear resistance, and should exhibit ductile behavior. The implant should require minimal bone resection and maintain the integrity of the joint.

O **What are the mechanisms of implant fixation?**

Implant fixation can be accomplished by cement (PMMA), direct interference fit, mechanical fasteners (such as screws or pins), adhesives and biological means.

○   **How is biological fixation achieved?**

Biological fixation is achieved by osteointegration. Osteointegration is the process by which bone attaches to a material or device. Osteointegration can be enhanced by two methods. The device can possess a textured or porous surface that will allow for the promotion of the growth of bone (osteoconduction). The device may also be coated with a material that plays an active role in promoting bone formation (osteoinduction). Such osteoinductive materials include hydroxyapatite and glass ceramics.

○   **What are some factors in the success of an implant?**

Implant success depends on the properties and biocompatibility of the implant material, the health of the recipient and the competency of the surgeon.

BIOMECHANICS

○ **What is the normal ankle joint motion during gait?**

The ankle is slightly dorsiflexed at heel contact, plantarflexes to achieve ground contact, dorsiflexes as the tibia moves over the foot, plantarflexes during propulsion and dorsiflexes during swing phase.

○ **What is ankle equinus?**

Ankle equinus is a sagittal plane deformity in which there is less than 10 degrees of available dorsiflexion at the ankle joint when the STJ is in neutral position and the midtarsal joint oblique axis is locked. Ankle equinus may be osseous or muscular.

○ **What are causes of ankle equinus?**

Osseus, morphology of articular surface; muscular; spastic paralysis (cerebral palsy, CVA); tonic spasm (e.g., secondary to painful heel); weak dorsiflexors, tight hamstrings; prolonged bed rest.

○ **Described the compensated equinus foot.**

The compensated equinus foot has excessive subtalar joint pronation to achieve dorsiflexion, unlocking of the midtarsal joint with midfoot collapse. It is associated with pronation induced pathologies and is very destructive.

○ **What happens in the uncompensated equinus foot type?**

The heel cannot touch the ground, resulting in a bouncy gait. There is excessive weightbearing on the forefoot leading to forefoot plantar callosities and clawing of the lesser digits, secondary hamstring contracture, supinator muscle contracture and proximal compensations such as genu recurvatum, abducted or adducted angle of gait, excessive knee flexion and hip flexion.

○ **What is the treatment for the equinus foot type?**

Heel lift to reduce strain; orthoses to control excessive pronation

○ **Where is the subtalar joint axis?**

16 degrees from the sagittal plane. 42 degrees from the transverse plane.

○ **What happens if the subtalar joint has a more vertical axis?**

There is more transverse plane motion.

○ **What happens if the subtalar joint has a more horizontal axis?**

There is more frontal plane motion.

○ **Describe the longitudinal axis and oblique axis of the midtarsal joint.**

The longitudinal axis is 15 degrees from the transverse plane and 9 degrees from the sagittal plane. The oblique axis is 52 degrees from the transverse plane and 57 degrees from the sagittal plane.

○   **What happens when the oblique axis of the midtarsal joint is high?**

When the oblique axis of the midtarsal joint is high, there will be large degrees of forefoot abduction with compensatory STJ and oblique axis MTJ pronation.

○   **What happens when the oblique axis of the midtarsal joint is low?**

There will be small degrees of forefoot adduction with compensatory STJ and oblique axis MTJ pronation.

○   **Describe the axis of motion of the ankle joint?**

The axis roughly aligns the tips of the malleoli; approximately 8 degrees to the transverse plane. The motion is mainly dorsiflexion with small amounts of abduction and plantarflexion with small amounts of adduction.

○   **What is the functional importance of ankle dorsiflexion?**

About 10 degrees of dorsiflexion is required for normal gait. Dorsiflexion is necessary to enable ground clearance during the swing phase of gait and to enable the tibia to move over the supporting foot during the stance phase of gait. The ankle joint acts as a sagittal plane pivot.

○   **Why is ankle plantarflexion important?**

Plantarflexion is important for generating power for active propulsion.

○   **What is the normal range of passive ankle dorsiflexion and plantarflexion?**

The normal range of passive ankle dorsiflexion is about 20 degrees and the normal range of passive ankle plantarflexion is about 50 degrees.

○   **What is the motion of the longitudinal axis of the midtarsal joint?**

The motion is pronation/supination, predominantly in the frontal plane.

○   **What is the motion of the oblique axis of the midtarsal joint?**

The motion is pronation/supination, predominantly in the sagittal and transverse plane

○   **How does the motion of the longitudinal axis of the midtarsal joint compare to the motion of the subtalar joint?**

The motions of the longitudinal axis of the midtarsal joint and the subtalar joint are opposites. In other words, when the STJ pronates the long axis of the MTJ supinates and vice versa. Supination of the long axis of the MTJ will unlock the midtarsal joint.

○   **What muscle with cause supination of the long axis of the MTJ?**

The tibialis anterior will cause supination of the long axis of the MTJ.

○   **What muscle will cause pronation of the oblique axis of the midtarsal joint?**

The peroneus longus will cause pronation (stability) of the oblique axis of the midtarsal joint. Ground reaction force will also cause pronation of the oblique axis of the MTJ.

○   **How does the subtalar joint influence the midtarsal joint?**

Subtalar joint pronation increases the range of motion available at the MTJ, which makes the foot flexible. Subtalar joint supination decreases the range of motion available at the MTJ which makes the foot rigid.

○   **What does recent research reveal about the midtarsal joint?**

The calcaneal cuboid joint and the talonavicular joint should be considered as 2 separate joints rather than a "midtarsal joint."

○   **What does the first ray consist of? Where is its axis?**

The first ray is a functional unit consisting of articulations between the 1st metatarrsal and medial cuneiform. The axis of the first ray is 45 degrees to the frontal and sagittal planes.

○   **What are the motions of the first ray?**

The motion is dorsiflexion with inversion and plantarflexion with eversion.

○   **What are the major muscles acting on the first ray?**

The major muscles acting on the first ray are the tibialis anterior and the peroneus longus.

○   **What are the motions of the first ray during gait?**

The first ray dorsiflexes when the foot pronates and plantarflexes during propulsion to enable normal MPJ dorsiflexion. The first ray should be parallel to the plane of the lesser rays. There should be equal amounts of dorsiflexion and plantarflexion.

○   **What can produce a plantarflexed first ray?**

Weak gastrocnemius (the foot will go into a rearfoot calcaneus position and the first ray will plantarflex to reach the ground); Hypertonicity of peroneus longus; weak tibialis anterior, cavus foot type.

○   **Describe the subtalar joint.**

The subtalar joint is formed by the posterior talocalcaneal joint and the acetabulum pedis lodging the talar head. The basic motion at the joint is that of supination (plantarflexion, adduction, inversion) or pronation (dorsiflexion, abduction, eversion). The subtalar joint motion is guided by the intrinsic ligaments, the interosseous talocalcaneal ligament of the tarsal canal and the cervical ligament. Further support is provided by the extrinsic ligaments: the calcaneofibular ligament and the tibiocalcaneal fascicle of the deltoid ligament.

○   **What is meant by the acetabulum pedis?**

The acetabulum pedis is formed by the calcaneal middle and anterior surfaces connected to the navicular articular surface by the inferior and superomedial calcaneonavicular ligaments. The acetabulum pedis has a variable volume capacity adapting to the position of the talar head.

○   **What is the passive range of motion of the subtalar joint?**

Average range of motion is about 20 to 30 degrees of inversion and about 5 to 10 degrees of eversion. However ranges of subtalar joint motion have been cited as from 10 degrees to 65 degrees total range of motion in various studies.

○ **Describe the hypermobile first ray.**

The hypermobile 1st ray has a high arch non-weightbearing, with the arch flattening out on weightbearing. Hyperkeratoses are likely to be present under the 2nd metatarsal head. The hypermobile plantarflexed first ray has been associated with juvenile HAV, Morton's neuroma, lesser toe deformities, plantar fasciitis and 1st met-cuneiform exostosis.

○ **Describe the rigid plantarflexed first ray.**

The rigid plantarflexed 1st ray is high arched off weightbearing and on weightbearing. The heel will be in the varus position when standing. Callosities will be present under the first and 5th metatarsal heads and under the lateral heel. The rigid plantarflexed 1st ray is associated with sesamoiditis, chronic inversion ankle sprains, tibial stress fracture, medial knee pain, and lower back pain.

○ **What is the cause of a dorsiflexed first ray?**

A dorsiflexed first ray, also called metatarsus primus elevatus, may be congenital or acquired. It may be caused by hypertonicity of the tibialis anterior muscle or weakness of the peroneus longus muscle. A dorsiflexed first ray may be associated with forefoot supinatus, dorsal jamming of the first MPJ and commonly associated with hallux limitus and rigidus.

○ **What is a flexible forefoot valgus deformity?**

A flexible forefoot valgus is one in which the MTJ has sufficient ROM to compensate for the everted forefoot.

○ **What is a rigid forefoot valgus?**

A rigid forefoot valgus is one in which there is inadequate MTJ ROM to compensate, so the STJ must supinate to bring the forefoot to the ground. The pathomechanics are that the forefoot is everted at forefoot loading, the long axis of the MTJ supinates and the STJ supinates.

○ **What happens to the foot with a rigid forefoot valgus?**

The foot is high arched nonweightbearing and weight bearing. The heel is inverted when standing. There is restricted motion of the MTJ and contracted lesser digits. There are calluses under the 1st and 5th metatarsal head and the lateral heel.

○ **What is the rigid forefoot valgus foot type associated with?**

The rigid forefoot valgus deformity is associated with sesamoiditis, chronic inversion ankle sprains, tibial stress fractures and medial knee pain, and low back pain.

○ **What is Blount's disease?**

A lateral slippage of the proximal tibial epiphysis.

○ **What is the pathomechanics of rearfoot varus according to Root biomechanics?**

The entire foot is in an inverted position. There is increased ground reaction force lateral to STJ at forefoot loading. The STJ pronates until the forefoot contacts the ground or the STJ range of motion is exhausted.

○   **What is a fully compensated rearfoot varus according to Root biomechanics?**

In a fully compensated rearfoot varus there is sufficient STJ ROM to bring the medial border of the forefoot to the ground. There is a very rapid contact phase of pronation. Pronation extends until heel lift. The forefoot will be hypermobile and there is overuse of the supinator musculature.

○   **What are signs and symptoms of rearfoot varus according to Root biomechanics?**

Medium arch height nonweightbearing with slight lowering of the arch on weightbearing; excessive lateral shoe wear, Haglund's deformity, tendinitis of the tibialis anterior, tibialis posterior, and long flexors; all pronation-induced pathologies.

○   **What happens in the uncompensated rearfoot varus according to Root biomechanics?**

The foot strikes the ground in an inverted position, (as it does normally), but there will be inadequate shock absorption from the STJ. There will be lateral instability. An acquired plantarflexed 1st ray may develop.

○   **Discuss orthotic management of rearfoot varus deformity.**

The purpose of orthotic management for rearfoot deformity is to eliminate STJ compensation and bring the ground up to the foot. This may be accomplished with a modified Root orthosis or Blake inverted orthosis.

○   **What is forefoot varus and its theoretical cause?**

Forefoot varus is a fixed, osseous congenital deformity in which the forefoot is inverted relative to the rearfoot when the subtalar joint is in the neutral position and the oblique axis of the MTJ is locked (pronated). However a true forefoot varus occurs only with a very few conditions such as talipes equinovarus (clubfoot). Most often, an inverted forefoot is actually forefoot supinatus and the supinatus is a compensatory inversion for rearfoot valgus upon standing. Theoretically forefoot varus was considered to be due to inadequate torsion of the head and neck of the talus during the fetal development, but this is not well supported and has shown to be incorrect in empirical studies.

○   **What is the pathomechanics of forefoot supinatus?**

The forefoot is inverted at forefoot loading. There is increased ground reaction force lateral to the STJ axis. The STJ pronates until the forefoot contacts the ground or STJ ROM is exhausted.

○   **Describe the fully compensated forefoot varus foot type.**

The fully compensated forefoot varus foot type consists of enough available STJ ROM to bring the entire forefoot in contact with the ground.

○   **Describe the partially compensated forefoot varus foot type.**

The partially compensated forefoot varus foot type has insufficient STJ ROM to bring the entire forefoot in contact with the ground.

○   **Describe the uncompensated forefoot varus foot type.**

In the uncompensated forefoot varus foot type, there is no STJ range of motion.

○   **What are the effects of the fully compensated forefoot varus foot type?**

The foot is mechanically unstable. There is breakdown of the MTJ as midfoot mobility increases. The angle of pull of the peroneus longus is altered, rendering the forefoot unstable. There is a decreased lever arm for the tibialis anterior. The angle of pull of the FDL becomes more oblique, leading to buckling of the toes.

○ What are some pathologies associated with the fully compensated forefoot varus foot type?

Virtually all pathologies associated with STJ pronation; medial tibial stress syndrome (shin splints), plantar fasciitis, tibialis posterior tendinitis, patello-femoral syndrome, lesser digital deformity, hallux abducto valgus.

○ What happens in the uncompensated forefoot varus foot type?

There is no pronation available at the STJ, therefore the forefoot is held in the inverted position through the gait cycle. The foot exhibits excessive lateral contact throughout stance phase, with very late stance phase weightbearing on the IPJ of the hallux as the limb moves forward. Hyperkeratosis may be present on the 5th MPJ and IPJ of the hallux. There may be excessive lateral shoe wear.

○ What is forefoot supinatus?

Forefoot supinatus is a triplanar, acquired soft tissue contracture of the forefoot in a supinated position around the longitudinal axis of the midtarsal joint caused by heel valgus. The heel valgus with subtalar joint pronation causes a compensatory supination around the longitudinal axis of the midtarsal joint.

○ What is the cause of forefoot supinatus?

Over time, the soft tissues will adapt to this position and the forefoot will appear inverted when placed in the subtalar joint neutral position. The peroneus longus stretches and elongates. The tibialis anterior shortens and contracts.

○ What are Newton's 3 laws?

The law of Inertia.
$F = ma$.
Action, Reaction.

○ What happens to the tibia when the foot supinates?

0 .44 degrees of outward rotation of the tibia occur for every degrees of supination of the foot. This indicates that the joints act together as a universal joint.

○ When is the adult gait pattern attained?

Between the ages of 7 and 9 years.

○ What are the major determinants of gait?

They are: (1) rotation of the pelvis about a vertical axis; (2) pelvic lateral list; (3) flexion of the knee during weight-bearing; (4) lateral displacement of the pelvis; (5 & 6) foot and knee motion.

○ What type of rotation occurs during gait?

Rotation in the transverse plane about a vertical axis occurs in the entire limb. The amount of rotation increases from the proximal to the distal segments. The rotation is internal during swing phase and the first 15 per cent of stance phase. Normally, during walking on level ground, the pelvis rotates an average of 8 degrees, the femur 15 degrees, and the tibia 19 degrees.

○ **When does external rotation occur during the gait cycle?**

From after 15% of stance phase until just after toe-off.

○ **Describe the trochlea of the talus.**

The trochlea of the talus is an average of 2.4 mm wider anteriorly than posteriorly. The trochlea is a portion of a cone. The base of the cone is toward the fibula with a longer radius laterally than medially; resulting in a larger anteroposterior displacement of the fibular than of the tibial malleolus when the foot is fixed on the floor and the leg moves over it.

○ **Describe the axis of the ankle joint.**

The axis of rotation of the ankle joint runs between the distal tips of the malleoli and is directed laterally and posteriorly when projected in the transverse plane. There is 20-30 degrees of external rotation in relation to the knee axis. The axis runs laterally and downward when projected on a coronal plane (average of 80 degree to the long axis of the tibia).

○ **Describe the motion of the ankle during gait.**

The motion of the ankle during gait is plantarflexion occurs from heel strike through the first 10 per cent of the cycle; then dorsiflexion occurs from heel-off to 40 percent of the cycle, at which time plantar flexion again occurs. During the swing phase the ankle is normally in dorsiflexion.

○ **What is the metatarsophalangeal break?**

The metatarsophalangeal break refers to the oblique axis through the second to fifth metatarsophalangeal joints. The angle between the break and the long axis of the foot varies from 54 to 73 degrees. During push-off, the hindfoot and midfoot are angle outward as the heel is inverted. The metatarsal break distributes weight on all the metatarsal heads rather than on the longest only.

○ **When during gait do the anterior compartment muscles act and what is their function?**

The anterior compartment muscles act primarily during the swing and early stance phase of gait and this action enables the foot to clear the ground during swing phase and then allows it to be placed gently on the ground after heel strike.

○ **When during gait do the calf muscles act and what is their function?**

The posterior or calf muscle act from midstance to toe-off. They aid the foot in propulsion.

○ **What happens to the subtalar joint during gait?**

The subtalar joint quickly everts 10 degrees within the first 8% of stance phase of gait. Once the forefoot contacts the floor, there is a slow reversal of motion, with inversion occurring as the heel rises during terminal stance.

○ **What muscle has the greatest inversion torque on the subtalar joint?**

The tibialis posterior has an 88% mechanical advantage over the tibialis anterior due to its larger cross section and greater lever arm. Although the tibialis posterior muscle has the longest inversion lever to the subtalar joint axis, the five times greater mass of the soleus muscle overcomes its shorter lever arm resulting in an inversion torque twice that of the tibialis posterior.

O   **How much subtalar joint rotation occurs during gait?**

6 degrees in normal feet and 12 degrees in flatfeet.

O   **What is the function of the intrinsic muscles of the foot?**

The intrinsic muscles function to help elevate the longitudinal arch of the foot and invert the calcaneus and act in conjunction with the plantar aponeurosis and gastrocsoleus muscle to carry out these functions.

O   **Where does the gastrosoleus muscle insert in relation to the subtalar joint axis?**

Medial to the subtalar joint axis.

O   **How much motion is present at the metatarsophalangeal joint in the normal foot?**

90 degrees of extension and 30 degrees of flexion.

O   **What is flexor stabilization?**

Flexor stabilization occurs during the stance phase of gait. The interossei muscles are overpowered by the flexor digitorum longus. The pull of the FDL is altered in the pronatory direction causing an increased pull on the distal phalanx of toes two through five resulting in hammer digits.

O   **What is extensor substitution?**

Extensor substitution occurs when the long extensor muscles overpower the lumbricales. The lumbricales act to stabilize the digits during swing phase and counteract the extensor digitorum longus pull. When the lumbricales are weakened a high-arched foot develops with hammer toes.

O   **What is the position of the subtalar joint during running?**

The subtalar joint is pronated during the entire running cycle.

O   **What is the ground reaction force during running?**

Depending on the runner's weight the ground reaction force is between three to eight times the body weight during running.

O   **When would the moment arm and the lever arm be the same?**

When the lever arm is perpendicular to the action line of the muscle.

O   **The action of a force applied to an object, which tends to rotate the object about an axis is known as:**

Moment.

O   **How many degrees of freedom would a rigid body moving through space without any restraints contain?**

6 degrees of freedom.

O   **What type lever is created by the forearm and elbow when picking up a glass from the table and what type of muscle action is created?**

Type 3 lever. The elbow is the pivot or axis. The forearm is the lever. The weight of the forearm and the glass is the resistance. The force of the biceps is the effort. The type of muscle force required to pick up a glass of water up off a table is concentric muscle force. Eccentric muscle force is used to place the glass back down on the table.

○ **What type of material requires very little stress to produce a significant amount of strain?**

A material, which is elastic.

○ **What type of material requires a sizable amount of stress to produce a small amount of strain?**

A material, which is rigid.

○ **How is the stiffness of a given material represented on the stress-strain curve?**

The slope of the curve in the elastic region.

○ **When a bone is subjected to three-point bending, where is the first place that fracture will occur?**

The tensile side.

○ **When the angle of pennation is 30 degrees, how much force is transmitted to the tendon?**

The angle of pennation is the angle that the muscle makes with the tendon in a pennated muscle. There are parallel muscles and pennated muscles. In parallel muscles the tendon is parallel and in series with the muscle, and therefore, 100% of the muscle force is transmitted into the tendon when the muscle contracts. In a pennated muscle the muscle fibers are at an angle with the tendon and the percentage of force that is transmitted by the muscle fibers into the tendon can be calculated by the angle of pennation X to Cosine of that angle. Therefore the angle of pennation is 30 degrees, the cosine of 30 degrees = .866. Therefore approximately 87% of the muscle force would be transmitted into the tendon for contraction when the muscle contracts. The remaining force is used for stabilizing and heat. When the angle of pennation reaches 60 degrees, only half of the force of the muscle reaches the tendon because the cosine of 60 degrees = .5. In nature the angle of pennation is usually very small and almost always acute.

○ **What happens when a ligament is loaded at a relatively high rate of loading?**

When a ligament is loaded at a relatively fast rate of loading, ligamentous failure occurs. When a ligament is loaded at a relatively slow rate of loading the ligament will avulse off the bone. This is true for tendons as well. For example in the styloid process fracture the peroneus brevis tendon is loaded at a relatively slow rate by inversion and plantarflexion until the tendon pulls the styloid process of the fifth metatarsal off the bone. All viscoelastic substances demonstrate this loading property.

○ **What is an anisotropic substance?**

An anisotropic substance has a grain, i.e., wood, bone, tendon, and therefore will demonstrate different properties depending upon the direction in which it is loaded. Metal has no grain and is an example of an isotropic substance and will demonstrate the same properties no matter which direction in which it is loaded.

○ **When standing up right in the anatomic position, where does the center of gravity pass with respect to the hips, knees, and ankles?**

The center of gravity passes posterior to the hips, anterior to the knee and anterior to the ankle.

○ **What is the coefficient of friction for joints in the human body?**

The coefficient of friction for joints in the human body is about .005.

○ **When do most ligaments fail?**

6-8% elongation.

○ **How does the ligamentum flavum differ from other ligaments in the body?**

It has a higher percentage of elastin. This results in great elasticity with virtually no plastic deformation. Therefore the ligamentum flavum has the mechanical properties of being both highly elastic and brittle. The human aorta has a very high content of elastin.

○ **What does friction depend upon and what is friction completely independent of?**

Friction is dependent upon type of surfaces in contact and the coefficient of friction. Friction is nearly independent of surface area and velocity.

○ **Why is it NOT possible to fully flex the wrist and make a fist?**

It is not possible to fully flex the wrist and make a fist at the same time because of active insufficiency. Active insufficiency occurs in 2-joint muscles and is caused by the inability of a 2-joint muscle to fully contract over both joints.

PUBLIC HEALTH
Community Medicine, Epidemiology, Biostatistics, And Geriatrics

PUBLIC HEALTH AND COMMUNITY MEDICINE

O **How do you define public health in general terms?**

Public health involves issues of physical, mental and social well-being and longevity.

O **As a discipline how would you characterize the components of public health?**

Public health is the art and science of: Preventing disease, prolonging life, and
promoting health and efficiency through organized community effort for sanitation, communicable disease, hygiene,
early diagnosis and preventive treatment, maintenance of health

O **What is the purpose of public health services?**

To prevent disease, to promote health, and to measure and evaluate the health status of populations

O **How do you define Community Health?**

That section of public health, which deals with issues of preventive medicine and epidemiology as they relate to
groups of people rather than individuals

O **How do you define Epidemiology?**

Epidemiology is the science of the study of health and disease in a population. It looks for the distribution and
determinants of health and disease in groups of people and it asks four questions who, where, when and how.

O **How do you define Biostatistics?**

Biostatistics is the study of the methods and procedures for collecting, summarizing and analyzing data about health
and disease and for making scientific inferences from such data.

O **How do you define Podiatric Public Health?**

Podiatric public health is that subset of public health which addresses the needs of the human foot and seeks to
prevent foot pathology, prolong optimum foot function, and promote foot health through primary, secondary and
tertiary preventive techniques, patient education and research.

O **How do you differentiate between primary, secondary and tertiary prevention?**

Primary Prevention: Efforts to prevent disease before it occurs. Secondary Prevention: Refers to screening for disease precursors in order to institute treatment before symptoms occur, Tertiary Prevention: Refers to efforts to arrest or retard the effects of a condition already established.

〇   **What are the principals of health education?**

Any combination of learning experiences designed to predispose, enable and reinforce voluntary adaptations of individuals or collective behavior conducive to health

〇   **What are the principals of health promotion?**

Health promotion, Health protection and Preventive health services.

〇   **Who provides the majority of public health services in the United States?**

The federal government provides the majority of public health services in the U.S..

〇   **How are public health services for State governments delivered?**

Each State constitution defines the responsibilities of the State government for the protection of the health of its citizens. There is no consistency how this is to be accomplished. As such, each state differs in how it manages the health concerns of its domain. Generally speaking, most states are divided into divisions of bureaus and provide for certain services in common. These components usually include; 1. Communicable disease control, 2. Vital statistics, 3. Environmental sanitation, 4. Maternal and child health, 5. Public health laboratory service, 6. Public health nursing, 7. Health education, 8. Local health services, 9. Mental hygiene, 10. Industrial hygiene 11. Administration.

〇   **How are public health services for local governments delivered?**

Additionally each State constitution demands that some of the responsibility for health rest with local governments. The following activities are considered basic for local governments; 1. Vital statistics, 2. Public health laboratory 3. Communicable disease control, 4. Environmental sanitation, 5. Maternal and child health, 6. Public health education.

〇   **What were the most common causes of death at the beginning of the 20th century and how does that compare to today's leading causes of death?**

In the early 20th century acute infectious communicable diseases were most common causes of death. Among the most common causes were: Tuberculosis, Pneumonia, Influenza, Smallpox, Typhus, and Typhoid. Today's leading causes of death: chronic degenerative diseases and include; 1. Heart disease 2. Cancer 3. Stroke 4. Accidents.

〇   **What are the three components of all disease?**

The etiology of all disease includes host, agent, and environmental components.

〇   **What are the determinants of disease?**

1.Inherited Disease
2. Environmental Effects such as Overcrowding, Air, water, noise and food pollution, Social conditions, Radiation hazards, Drugs: (Over the counter, prescription and illicit medications), Poisons: (There are three classifications of poisons; 1. irritant, 2. Neurotoxins and 3. Hemotoxins.)
3. Infectious process: Increasingly resistant strains of bacteria are evolving and diseases such as tuberculosis which had been under control are re - emerging.
4. Nutritional deficiency: obesity, bulimia, anorexia

5. Metabolic disturbances: Diabetes continues to be the most common metabolic disorder and creates significant lower extremity morbidity and mortality.

6. Allergic disturbances - foods can cause allergic gastroenteropathy and may cause atopic dermatitis, asthma, anaphylaxis, and urticaria or angioedema. Allergic reactions to drugs are commonly urticaria and anaphylaxis.

7. Aging and degenerative processes - aging is characterized by the progressive constriction of each organ system's homeostatic reserve. In the absence of disease, the decline in homeostatic reserve should cause no symptoms and impose no restrictions on activities of daily living regardless of age. As people age they are at a higher risk of suffering from disease, disability, and drug side effects.

8. Accidental injuries: Males aged 16-35 are at especially high risk for serious injury and death from accidents and violence. Having a gun in the home increases the likelihood of homicide by 2.7-fold and of suicide by 5-fold.

9. Cancer and neoplasm's - cigarette smoking is the most important preventable cause of cancer. Primary prevention of skin cancer consists of restricting exposure to UV light. Generally accepted techniques exist of secondary prevention of cancers of the breast, colon, and cervix through cancer screening procedures.

○   **How are the risk categories for health care workers defined?**

Category 1 - frequent, direct contact with blood and body fluids - phlebotomists, surgeons, laboratory technicians, sanitation workers.
Category 2 - infrequent - x-ray technician, EKG technician.
Category 3 - seldom – receptionist.

○   **What are the Universal Infections Control Procedures?**

Hand washing.
Barriers, gloves, gowns, sleeves, aprons, masks, goggles, face shields.
Needles and sharps, disposed in puncture proof container, do not re-cap needles, remove blades with hemostat.
Fluid spills, chemical germicides, hospital disinfectants.
Specimens, sealed containers f. Instruments, standard sterilization and disinfection procedures are adequate, cold sterile is OK for non-invasive instruments, autoclave instruments which invade tissue or vascular system.

○   **What are the agencies involved in health issues and their respective percent of the federal health care budget?**

1. Department of Health and Human Services - 75%
2. Veterans Administration - 10%
3. Department of Defense - 7%
4. Other - 1.5%
       a-Department of Agriculture
            1. Food inspection
            2. Food stamp program
       b-Environmental Protection agency
       c-Department of Labor
            1. Occupational Safety and Health Act (OSHA) - General responsibility to protect employees against both safety and health hazards.
            2. National Institute for Occupational Safety and Health (NIOSH) - This is a research body which develops recommendations occupational and safety stands to OSHA.

○   **Which is the largest governmental agency involved in health care and when was it formed?**

The Department of Health and Human Services is the largest federal government department by budget and number of employees. It replaced the Department of Health Education and Welfare in 1979 which split into Department of Education and DHHS.

○   **What are the major components of the DHHS?**

Office of Human Development.
Public Health Service.
Health Care Financing Administration.
Social Security Administration.

O   **What are the two principal HEALTH agencies of DHHS:**

Health Care Financing Administration (HCFA)
United States Public Health Service

O   **How does the Health Care Financing Administration (HCFA) function?**

Primary function is to run the government's two major treatment services, Medicare and Medicaid. It oversees the financing of and manages, directs and administers Medicare and Medicaid

O   **What major health programs were provided for in the 1965 Amendments To The Social Security Act?**

Established MEDICARE in TITLE 18, and established MEDICAID in TITLE 19

O   **What did the 1967 Amendments To The Social Security Act provide for with respect to podiatric medicine?**

Added Podiatrists to the list of Physicians, added Podiatric care as a covered service but excluded services including orthotics and treatment for subluxations and "Routine foot care" which it defined as corns, calluses, nails and other routine hygienic care.

O   **What are the benefits provided for in Medicare Title 18?**

Provides health care for the elderly, blind and disabled.
        Part A (involuntary)
                -inpatient services $520.00 deductible
                -extended care services
                -home health services
                -outpatient diagnostic services
        Part B (voluntary with a monthly premium paid by the patient)
                -Doctors fees, $100.00 deductible, pays 80% of Approved costs, Additional 20% due from patient

O   **What are the benefits provided in Medicaid: Title 19?**

Provides medical care for indigent populations, funded by the federal and state governments, Arizona does not provide a Medicaid program for its residents. Programs inlcude: Aid to the Aged, aid to Families of Dependent Children, aid to the Blind, aid to the Disabled. It is called Medicaid in 49 states and called MediCal in California

O   **What are the major components of the Public Health Service?**

Alcohol, Drug Abuse and Mental Health Administration, defined by its name.

Centers for Disease Control and Prevention. Functions to prevent and control communicable disease, to direct foreign and interstate quarantine operations and to improve the performance of clinical laboratories. Serves as the national focus for developing and applying disease prevention and control, environmental health and health promotion and health education activities designed to improve the health of the people of the U.S.

Food and Drug Administration

The FDA is a monitoring agency which reviews products in order to protect the public against hazards of electronic and radiological products, assuring the safety and efficacy of drugs, medical devices and biologicals, assuring the purity of food, regulating the production of animal feeds and drugs and assuring safety of cosmetics

Health Resources and Services Administration

HRSA operates several direct health care and support services. It supports health sciences education, health planing, health facility construction, The Community Health Centers program, The national Health Services Corps and Health Maintenance Organization development.

National Institutes of Health

The NIH is the major national force in biomedical research
National Cancer Institute
National Heart, Lung, and Blood Institute
National Library of Medicine - serves as the Nation's principal source of medical information provided by medical library services and on-line bibliographic searching capabilities, such as MEDLINE, TOXLINE, and others.
National Institute of Diabetes and Digestive and Kidney Diseases
National Institute of Allergy and Infectious Diseases
National Institute of Child Health and Human Development
National Institute on Deafness and Other Communication Disorders
National Institute of Dental Research
National Institute of Environmental Health Sciences
National Institute of General Medical Sciences
National Institute of Neurological Disorders and Stroke
National Eye Institute
National Institute on Aging
National Institute of Alcohol Abuse and Alcoholism
National Institute of Arthritis and Musculoskeletal and Skin Diseases
National Institute on Drug Abuse
National Institute of Mental Health
Clinical Center - designed to provide a setting in which scientist working in the Clinic's laboratories can work in close proximity with clinicians caring for patients to collaborate on problems of mutual concern.
Fogarty International Center - promotes development of science internationally as it relates to health.
National Center of Human Genome Research
National Center for Nursing Research
Division of Computer Research and Technology
National Center for Research Resources
Division of Research Grants

Office of the Assistant Secretary of Health

-founded in 1985
-Offices of Disease Prevention and Health Promotion
-Population Affairs
-Smoking and Health
-International Health
-Presidents Council on Physical Fitness and Sports
-National Centers for Health Statistics
-National Centers for Health Services Research

O   **What are the components of the Health Resources and Services Administration (HRSA)?**

Bureau of Health Professions - provides national leadership in coordinating, evaluating, and supporting the development and utilization of the Nation's health personnel. Provides grants for health professions, Funds regional centers that provide educational services and training, Administers several loan programs supporting student training and serves as a focus for technical assistance.

Indian Health Service - provides a comprehensive health services delivery system for American Indians and Alaska Natives with opportunity for maximum tribal involvement in developing and managing programs to meet their health needs.

Bureau of Resources and Development - develops, coordinates, administers, directs, monitors, and supports Federal policy and programs pertaining to health care facilities; national network associated with organ donations and transplants, and activities related to AIDS.

Bureau of Primary Health Care - serves to ensure the availability and delivery of health care services in health professional shortage areas, to medically underserved populations, and to those with special needs. Provides project grants, administers the National Health Service Corps Bureau and National Health Service Corps Scholarship and Loan Repayment Programs.

Maternal and Child Health Bureau - addresses the full spectrum of primary, secondary, and tertiary care services and related activities conducted in the public and private sector which impact upon maternal and child health.

○ **How does the Department of Veterans Health Affairs provide public health?**

Provides health services - provides hospital, nursing home, and domiciliary care, and outpatient medical and dental care to eligible veterans of military service in the Armed Forces.

○ **What are the benefits provided to America's Veterans by the VA?**

Compensation and Pension - claims for disability compensation and pension, adaptive equipment, adapted housing, survivors' claims for death compensation, dependency and indemnity compensation, death pension, burial and lot allowance claims.

Education - responsible for the Montgomery GI Bill, the Post Vietnam Era Veterans' Educational Assistance Program, the Survivors' and Dependents' Educational Assistance Program, school approvals and compliance surveys.

Loan Guaranty - establish the eligibility of veterans for the program, passing on the ability of a veteran to repay a loan and the credit risk, and under certain conditions, guaranteed refinancing loans.

Insurance - life insurance operations are for the benefit of service members, veterans, and their beneficiaries. Includes complete maintenance of individual accounts, underwriting functions, and life and death insurance claims awards, and any other insurance-related transactions.

Medical Care including Podiatric Services - The V.A. established Podiatric services in 1976.

○ **What is the Department Of Defense role in health care?**

The DOD is involved in health care. Its chief medical officer is responsible for both treatment services and public health services for their installation. DOD operates 170 hospital of which 129 are in the U.S.

○ **What role does the Department of Agriculture play in public health?**

USDA is responsible for human, animal and plant health in the U.S. Active programs include: National School Lunch Program and Food Stamp Program

○ **What role does the Environmental Protection Agency play in public health?**

Independent federal agency which control air and water quality and pollution control, solid waste disposal control, pesticide regulation, radiation hazard control, noise reduction and toxic substances.

○   **What is the difference between a Professional Standards Review Organization (PSRO) and a Professional Review Organization (PRO)? How does a PRO function?**

Professional Standards Review Organizations were established in 1972 to Review:
  * Hospital standards
  * Length of stay review
  * Medical care studies
  * Recommend denials for payment]
Professional Review Organizations (PRO) came about when a 1982 law repealed PSRO and established PRO to:
  * Determine medical necessity
  * Quality of care
  * Appropriateness of care
  * Tied to DRG's

STATISTICS AND EPIDEMIOLOGY

○   **What are the most common types of clinical studies?**

Prospective: follows a group of patients forward in time to determine an issue of disease.
Retrospective: begins at the present time and looks backward to identify data of interest.
Descriptive: provides a specific snapshot of various demographic and clinical data in a sample population.
Observational: clinical studies where the investigator is unable to manipulate the primary variables. Observations are made from observation of reality.
Interventional: experiments where the investigator is able to manipulate the variables to test a specific hypothesis.
Clinical Trials: prospective and interventional.
Case Controlled Studies: Retrospective and observational.
Cohort Studies: may be retrospective or prospective, descriptive, observational or interventional.

○   **What are the most common biostatistical rates and how are they used?**

Prevalence Rate

$$\frac{\text{All cases of a given disease at a given time}}{\text{Estimated population}} \times 1000$$

Example: In a population of 200 there are 25 people with tinea pedis on January 1, 1996 the prevalence rate for tinea pedis would be 25/200 x 1000 = 12.5/1000

Incidence

$$\frac{\text{New Cases of Disease Per Unit Time}}{\text{Estimated Population}} \times 10$$

Example: In a population of 200 persons 12 people present with onychocryptosis in the month of January 1996 and 15 persons present in the month of February. The incidence rate for January would be 12/200 x 1000 = 60/1000. The incidence rate for February would be 15/200 x 1000 = 75/1000.

False Positive

$$\frac{\text{Persons Without the Disease Positive to Test}}{\text{Total Non - Diseased}} \times 100$$

False Negative

$$\frac{\text{Persons With Disease Negative to Test}}{\text{Total Diseased}} \times 100$$

Sensitivity: True Positive

$$\frac{\text{Number of Positives With Disease}}{\text{Total With Disease Present}} \times 100$$

Specificity: True Negative

$$\frac{\text{Number of Negative Without Disease}}{\text{Number Who Do Not Have Disease}} \times 100$$

Example: In a test population of 200 persons 75 persons tested positive and 125 tested negative for fungus infection using the KOH test. DTM culture testing revealed that of the 75 testing positive 50 actually had a fungus and 25 did not. In addition, of the 125 testing negative 15 actually had fungus and 110 did not.

The False Positives in this scenario is calculated $25/135 \times 100 = 18.5/100$
The False Negative in this scenario is calculated $15/65 \times 100 = 23/100$
The Sensitivity or True Positive is calculated $50/65 \times 100 = 77$
The Specificity or True Negative is calculated $110/135 \times 100 = 81$

O   **What are Measures of Central Tendency and how are they used to evaluate information?**

Measures of central tendency are used as summary measures to describe data.

Mean - Numerical average
Median - Middle most value in a set of numbers or values
Mode - Most frequently occurring value or number.

O   **What are Measures of Variability and how are they used to evaluate information?**

Measures of variability are used as methods to measure scatter or dispersion.

Range - The largest number or value minus the smallest number.
Standard Deviation - Most frequently used measure of variability, in a normal curve.
         2 Standard Deviations = a central range in which 95.45% of the measurements lie.
         3 Standard deviations = a central range in which 99% of the measurement lie.

O   **What does the term "Statistical Significance" mean?**

A result, which cannot be explained by chance

O   **What is a Null Hypothesis?**

Negative reasoning that Treatment A is no different than treatment B. If accepted in the study, then there is insufficient evidence to prove otherwise.

O   **What is the Chi Squared test?**

Demonstrates whether or not there is an association between a factor or attribute and an outcome.

GERIATRICS

○ **What is Interdisciplinary Geriatric Assessment and how is it accomplished?**

Interdisciplinary geriatric assessment is a comprehensive method of evaluation of aging patients. It consists of a core team of geriatrician, nurse practitioner, social worker and in some cases a psychologist. They provide the geriatric patient with the necessary interdisciplinary approach for healthcare of the elderly patient.

○ **What role does the core team play in the assessments?**

Geriatrician - to assess the changes of normal aging as distinguished from disease effects. Nurse practitioner - to assess the functional capacity of the patient by assessing the patient's ability to perform the basic activities of daily living (ADL's) which are needed for self-care. The less incapacitated patient should be evaluated for instrumental activities of daily living (IADL's) which include shopping, money management, cooking, etc. Assessment is necessary to determine the patient's level of independence. Social worker - to assess the ability of the family, friends, and community agencies to provide those supports that will allow the patient to remain at home. Financial and family problems are often elucidated by the social worker.

○ **How would you describe the assessment process?**

Evaluation: the core team performs a comprehensive evaluation.
Prioritizing medical, nursing and social issues.
Coordinating referrals and management.

○ **Which professions are considered the primary consultants to the core team?**

Audiology, clinical psychology, dentistry, nutrition, occupational therapy, physical therapy, Podiatry, speech pathology, clergy

○ **Which professions are considered secondary consultants?**

Neurology, ophthalmology, orthopedics, physiatry, surgery, urology

○ **What are the signs and symptoms of progressive dementia syndromes (Alzheimer's disease)**

Early in the disease process problems of memory, particularly recent or short-term memory, mild personality changes, tendency to withdraw from social interactions may be evident. Later in the disease problems in abstract thinking or in intellectual functioning develop. Further disturbances in behavior and appearance may be seen, such as agitation, irritability, quarrelsomeness, and diminishing ability to dress appropriately. Patient may appear to be confused or disoriented about the month or year, patient may begin to wander, be unable to engage in conversation, seem inattentive and erratic in mood, appear uncooperative, and lose bladder and bowel control. By the end of the disease the patients will be incapable of caring for themselves.

○ **How are progressive dementia syndromes diagnosed?**

Clinical presentation with dementia, significant loss of intellectual abilities; insidious onset of symptoms, subtly progressive and irreversible course with documented deterioration over time; and exclusion of all other specific causes of dementia by history, physical examination, laboratory tests, psychometric, and other tests. There are no specific clinical tests or findings that are unique to Alzheimer's disease.

○ **What are the interventional strategies for progressive dementia syndromes?**

These can involve support from the family, the help of a homemaker or other aide in the home, employment of behavioral therapies, and the use of medication. Sources can include family support groups such as Alzheimer's

Association (AA), professional consultations for the patient and family with a mental health specialist, and a variety of community programs such as day or respite care. Every state has an agency on aging that provides information on services and programs, such as local Office on Aging, a Community Mental Health Center or local Medical Society, or a local chapter of AA.

O   **What are some examples of reversible forms of dementia?**

Reversible dementia syndromes (Side effects of medication, Substance abuse, Metabolic disorders, Circulatory disorders, Neurological disorders, Infections, Trauma, Toxins, Tumors).

O   **What are the signs and symptoms of reversible forms of dementia?**

Forgetfulness in the absence of depression and inattentiveness, significant cognitive impairment, and changes in emotional behavior or personality.

O   **How are reversible forms of dementia diagnosed?**

Based on history and on the physical and mental status examinations- supplemented by careful review of the patient's medication list and alcohol intake- and by laboratory investigations to exclude other causes of cognitive impairment.

O   **What are some examples of interventional strategies for reversible forms of dementia?**

With acknowledgment of changes in the patient's behavior or cognitive function, medical treatment is necessary to search and correct the treatable factor influencing the onset of the dementia. Treatment should include discontinuation of nonessential medications, treat coexisting medical and psychiatric problems, and family assistance in dealing with the condition.

O   **What are normal age related changes?**

In general, elderly patients experience an increase in body fat with decrease in total body water. With aging, Eyes and Ears related changes are: presbyopia, lens opacification, and decrease in high-frequency acuity; Endocrine related changes are: impaired glucose, decreased vitamin D absorption and activation and decreased testosterone; Respiratory related changes: decreased lung elasticity and increased chest wall stiffness; cardiovascular related changes: increased systolic blood pressure and decreased arterial compliance; Gastrointestinal related changes: decreased gastric acidity, decreased colonic motility, decreased anorectal function, and decreased hepatic function; Hematological and immune systems related changes: decreased T-cell function and increased autoantibodies; Renal related changes: decreased GFR and decreased urine concentration-dilution; Genitourinary related changes: vaginal and urethral mucosal atrophy and prostate enlargement; Musculoskeletal related changes: decreased lean body mass and decreased bone density; and Nervous system related changes: brain atrophy, decreased stage 4 sleep, and decreased brain catechol and dopaminergic synthesis.

O   **What are considered abnormal age related changes?**

Those changes caused by disease, not by age. These abnormal changes include: obesity, anorexia, blindness, deafness, diabetes mellitus, thyroid dysfunction, impotence, osteoporosis, osteomalacia, dyspnea, hypoxia, syncope, heart failure, heart block, cirrhosis, fecal impaction, fecal incontinence, anemia, autoimmune disease, symptomatic UTI, urinary incontinence, urinary retention, hip fracture, dementia, depression, Parkinson's disease, sleep apnea. and falls.

CANCER AND TUMORS

❍ **What bone tumor would be likely in a teenage male with night pain relieved by aspirin?**

Osteoid osteoma.

❍ **An expansile, oval, lucent lesion in the proximal phalanx of a thirty-five-year-old female is most likely a (an)?**

Enchondroma.

❍ **Do large or small lesions typically characterize malignant bone tumors?**

Large.

❍ **"Onion skin" changes in the periosteum are typical of what bone tumor?**

Ewing's sarcoma.

❍ **Why are malignant bone tumors unlikely to be expansile?**

They grow too fast.

❍ **"Ground Glass" tumor matrix is often seen with what bone tumor?**

Fibrous Dysplasia.

❍ **Why do pathological fractures and rickets-like bowing occur in fibrous dysplasia patients?**

Normal osseous tissue is replaced by fibrous tissue thus weakening the bone(s).

❍ **Malignant tumors are often characterized by intense periosteal reactions. List four such descriptive reactions.**

"Hair on end," "sunburst," Codman's triangle, "onion skin."

❍ **List three patterns of osseous destruction from bone tumors in ascending order of aggressivenes**

Geographic, moth-eaten, and permeative.

❍ **If a soft tissue mass is associated with an osseous tumor, this indicates a tendency for the tumor to be benign or malignant?**

Malignant.

❍ **To prevent recurrence on removing an osteoid osteoma surgically, the surgeon must do what?**

Excise central lucent nidus.

○   **Can an enchondroma convert to a malignant lesion and, if so, what?**

Yes, chondrosarcoma.

○   **A disease manifested by multiple enchondromas is called**

Ollier's disease.

○   **Maffuci's disease is characterized by**

Multiple enchondromas and hemangiomatosis.

○   **Name four benign bone tumors that can convert to a malignant one.**

Osteochondroma, enchondroma, giant cell, and fibrous dysplasia.

○   **Regarding the clinical/radiographic/laboratory presentation, list ten commonalities for osteogenic sarcoma and osteomyelitis.**

Malaise ("sick" patient), calor at the site, erythema at the site, tenderness at the site, edema at the site, possible fever, bony destruction on radiograph, Codman's triangle on radiograph, positive bone scan and increased WBCs.

○   **Describe the patient profile for chondrosarcoma.**

Male in his fifties.

○   **A pathological fracture of a unicameral bone cyst can result in what radiographic finding?**

The fallen fragment sign.

○   **The metastatic lesion most commonly found distal to the knees and elbows results from what primary tumor?**

Lung cancer.

○   **List three findings associated with McCune-Albright's syndrome.**

Fibrous dysplasia, Café au Lait spots ("coast of Maine"), and precocious puberty.

○   **Why do aggressive and malignant primary bone tumors most frequently occur in the distal femur, proximal tibia, proximal femur and proximal humerus?**

These are the regions of the greatest longitudinal bone growth.

○   **Name a malignant primary bone tumor that may be found in the diaphysis.**

Ewing's sarcoma.

○   **Name three classifications of malignant lesions.**

Mesenchymal, myeloproliferative and metastatic.

○   **Why is osteoid osteoma pain worse at night?**

Diurnal production of prostaglandins.

○ **Define synovial chondromatosis**

A benign condition in which metaplasia of synovial tissue results in the production of intra-articular loose bodies.

○ **What is the difference between a nonossifying fibroma and a fibrous cortical defect?**

Size. The fibrous cortical defect is less than 4 cm and the nonossifying fibroma is greater than 4 cm.

○ **With regards to bone tumors, what do the terms monostotic and polyostotic refer to?**

Monostotic—One bone is involved; Polyostotic—greater than one bone is involved.

○ **Fibrous dysplasia leading to a varus deformity of the femur is also known as**

The shepherd's crook deformity.

○ **Name the most common primary malignant bone tumor and the most common benign bone tumor.**

Multiple myeloma and osteochondroma, respectively.

○ **What is another name for primary non-Hodgkin's lymphoma (NHL)?**

Reticulum sarcoma of the bone.

○ **Multiple myeloma is a malignant tumor of what?**

Plasma cells.

○ **Histologically speaking, plantar fibromatosis may resemble what malignant condition?**

Fibrosarcoma.

○ **Knuckle pads on the toes, leukonychia and impaired hearing form what syndrome?**

Bart-Pumphrey syndrome.

○ **Periungual fibromas may be associated with what disease:**

Tuberous sclerosis.

○ **A giant cell tumor involving the joint space is called**

Pigmented villonodular synovitis.

○ **What is the most common malignant soft tissue tumor in patients from 0-25 years of age?**

Rhabdomyosarcoma.

○ **Name four types of Kaposi's sarcoma**

Classic, African, immuno-suppressed patient, and AIDS-related.

○   **The "rodent ulcer" is associated with what condition?**

Basal cell carcinoma.

○   **Which is the most aggressive condition: Squamous cell carcinoma or basal cell carcinoma?**

Squamous cell carcinoma.

○   **What is Bowen's disease?**

Squamous cell carcinoma in situ.

○   **What type of melanoma is most commonly seen in Blacks and on the soles of the feet?**

Acral lentiginous melanoma.

○   **What type of melanoma is most aggressive—nodular or superficial spreading?**

Nodular.

○   **Name the two classification systems for melanoma that grade level of invasion and tumor thickness respectively.**

Clark's and Breslow's.

○   **What is Dupuytren's exostosis?**

Subungual osteochondroma.

○   **What is mycosis fungoides?**

Cutaneous T-cell lymphoma.

○   **In assessing suspicious pigmented lesions, what does A, B, C, D, and E refer to?**

A—asymmetry.
B—border.
C—color.
D—diameter.
E—elevation.

○   **What is the most common type of melanoma?**

Superficial spreading.

○   **What is the most common cancer in man?**

Basal cell carcinoma.

○   **Osteosarcoma is chiefly a disease of individuals of less than 20 years of age. What pre-existing condition can result in a secondary peak in incidence for older adults?**

Paget's disease.

❍ **What is the most common site for metastases of osteosarcoma?**

Lung.

❍ **What malignant tumor are patients with Ollier's disease at risk for?**

Chondrosarcoma.

❍ **Which classification of leukemia predominates in childhood? In the aged?**

Acute lymphoblastic leukemia (ALL) and chronic lymphocytic leukemia (CLL), respectively.

❍ **What is the most likely diagnosis for a lesion overlying the distal interphalangeal joint that appears to be a "ganglion of the skin"?**

Mucoid cysts (myxoid cysts).

❍ **What gender is most afflicted with plantar fibromatosis?**

Male.

❍ **In removing the plantar fascia for multiple plantar fibromatosis, special care must be taken with what vital structure?**

Medial plantar nerve.

❍ **Fibrosarcoma has a predilection for upper or lower extremities?**

Lower.

❍ **How does a neurofibroma differ from a neurilemmoma regarding axons?**

In a neurofibroma, axons course through the tumor whereas axons are pushed to the side by the neurilemmoma (schwannoma).

❍ **What is the most implicated factor in pathogenesis of basal cell carcinoma?**

Exposure of skin to ultraviolet light (UVL).

❍ **When are the majority of hemangiomas first noticed?**

At birth.

❍ **Pyogenic granuloma of the nail bed is frequently confused with what?**

Proud flesh.

❍ **What is a Popoff tumor?**

A glomus tumor.

❍ **List the four descriptive terms used to describe a bone tumor's position in a bone.**

Central, eccentric, cortical and parosteal.

❍   **Name three benign bone tumors that can have a "soap bubble" matrix?**

Aneurysmal bone cyst, giant cell tumor, chondromyxoid fibroma.

❍   **What bone tumor can resemble a miniature physeal region?**

Osteochondroma.

❍   **A bone tumor in which the trabecular pattern usually runs perpendicular to the axis of the long bone with which it is associated?**

Osteochondroma.

❍   **Name a bone tumor characterized by "chicken wire" calcification.**

Chondroblastoma.

❍   **What are the two most common bones of the foot affected by primary bone tumors?**

The calcaneus and the metatarsals.

CAVUS FOOT

○ **Pes cavus is primarily of deformity in which body plane?**

Sagittal plane.

○ **How is pes cavus deformity classified?**

Pes cavus is classified as anterior cavus, posterior cavus, or a combination. The deformity is further classified as flexible (positional - reduces with weight bearing) or rigid (structural -does not reduce with weight bearing). Anterior cavus can be further divided based on the apex of the deformity – metatarsal cavus (occurring at Lisfranc's joint), lesser tarsal cavus (occurring over lesser tarsal bones), forefoot cavus (occurring at Chopart's joint), and combined anterior cavus (excessive plantarflexion occurring at two or more of the areas mentioned).

○ **What does anterior cavus mean?**

The forefoot or any of its components is plantarflexed on the rearfoot.

○ **What does posterior cavus mean?**

The rearfoot is excessively dorsiflexed on the forefoot.

○ **What are the etiologies of pes cavus deformity?**

Congenital, acquired, or idiopathic.

○ **When examining a patient with a pes cavus deformity, which part of the exam deserves special attention? Why?**

The neurologic exam deserves special attention because there is a high correlation between neuromuscular disorders and pes cavus.

○ **What are some congenital etiologies of cavus deformity?**

Myelodysplasia, myelomeningocele, spina bifida, Charcot-Marie-Tooth disease, Friedreich's ataxia, Roussy-Levy syndrome, cerebral palsy, muscular dystrophy, clubfoot, syphilis, and hypertrophic interstitial neuropathy (Dejerine-Sottas syndrome).

○ **What are some acquired etiologies of pes cavus?**

Poliomyelitis, dystonia musculorum deformans, spinal cord tumors, trauma, infection, Lederhose disease, hysteria, and stroke.

○ **What are idiopathic etiologies of pes cavus?**

Those, which are inherent to the foot, that create the sagittal plane deformity of pes cavus.

○ **How does the foot compensate for a cavus deformity?**

Retraction of the toes occurs when there is overpowering or unopposed pull by the extensor tendons. This occurs at rest and is exaggerated during swing phase leading to a fixed deformity. It may also be the result of extensor substitution. As a result of retrograde force from the digits, the metatarsal heads become more plantargrade. The extensor apparatus gains the mechanical advantage and the anterior cavus increases. Forefoot reduction of the flexible anterior cavus occurs with ground reactive force. This is absorbed at the midtarsal level and if fully absorbed the foot will appear normal during weight bearing. If it cannot fully absorb the sagittal plane motion necessary to reduce the foot (because the deformity is rigid) then the ankle will dorsiflex. This compensation for the rigid anterior cavus leads to a pseudo equinus as the talus becomes maximally dorsiflexed and the calcaneal inclination angle increases. This high calcaneal inclination has traditionally been described as a posterior cavus. This would rarely exist as the primary deforming force. The subtalar joint does not compensate for sagittal plane anterior cavus deformity.

○   **What is the relationship between forefoot varus and cavus foot?**

Forefoot varus can be thought of as lateral column or the 4th and 5th metatarsals and cuboid being plantarflexed on the rearfoot. This compensates with subtalar pronation and has the appearance of a high arched pronated foot.

○   **What is the relationship between forefoot valgus and cavus foot?**

Forefoot valgus can be thought of as medial column or the 1st, 2nd, 3rd metatarsals, the cuneiforms, and navicular being plantarflexed in respect to the rearfoot. This compensates with subtalar or midtarsal supination. In subtalar supination the foot functions as a high arched foot with no pronation and little shock absorbing capability. Lateral ankle instability may result due to the inverted position of the calcaneus. With midtarsal supination the joint becomes unlocked, making the forefoot unstable, which can lead to subtalar pronation.

○   **What is the relationship between plantarflexed first ray and cavus foot?**

Plantarflexed first ray can exist as a) plantarflexed 1st metatarsal with metatarsals 1-5 varus. In this case, metatarsals 2-5 must be more varus than that of 1-5. Compensation for this foot type will be similar to that for forefoot varus except there will be more pressure on metatarsal heads 1 and 5 or 1 and 4, and 5. An anterior cavus in this type of plantarflexed 1st ray will be a high-arch pronated foot with increased pressure on the weight bearing metatarsals. b) plantarflexed 1st metatarsal and varus attitude of metatarsal 2-5. This foot type may function relatively normally but with more pressure on metatarsals 1 and 5, or 1 and 4, and 5. Little pressure will be borne on the 2nd and 3rd metatarsal heads. An anterior cavus will increase the pressure on these metatarsals. c) valgus position of metatarsals 1-5. Compensation for this type of plantarflexed 1st ray will be similar that for forefoot valgus except there will be increased pressure on metatarsal 1 and 5 or 1 and 4, and 5. An anterior cavus in this type of plantarflexed 1st ray will cause additional pressure on the weight bearing metatarsals.

○   **What is the relationship between metatarsus adductus and cavus foot?**

Metatarsus adductus is a structural deformity in which the metatarsals are excessively adducted in relation to the lesser tarsus at Lisfranc's joint. This deformity usually leads to an adducted gait with pronation being the compensation, thus unlocking the MTJ and allowing abduction at Chopart's joint, which masks the adduction at Lisfranc's joint. A skewfoot, or "Z" shaped foot results. When anterior cavus is superimposed on the met adductus foot, the ground reactive forces are increased adding to the severity of the deformity.

○   **What is pseudo equinus?**

Pseudo equinus is not a true limitation of ankle dorsiflexion at the ankle joint but is rather the condition that exists when available ankle dorsiflexion potential is used up in order to compensate for an anterior equinus. Thus the ankle functions as if there is a limitation of ankle dorsiflexion.

○   **What is the relationship between rearfoot equinus and cavus foot?**

Rearfoot equinus includes those deformities, which restrict ankle dorsiflexion. These include gastrocnemius, gastrosoleus, osseous, and pseudo equinus. These deformities compensate by early heel-off or lack of heel contact. Compensation may also lead to subtalar pronation with or without early heel-off, steppage gait, genu recurvatum, hip flexion, or flexed knee gait.

○ **What is the relationship between rearfoot varus and cavus foot?**

Rearfoot varus is a deformity in which the posterior aspect of the calcaneus is inverted relative to the perpendicular when the subtalar joint is in the neutral position and the patient is in the angle and base of gait. Compensation occurs by eversion to the perpendicular to allow the foot to contact the ground. Lateral ankle instability may result when this condition cannot fully compensate.

○ **What type of surgical procedures may be indicated for pes cavus in the face of progressive neuromuscular disease?**

Joint stabilization or fusion procedures may be indicated when deformities are progressive.

○ **When evaluating the weight bearing rearfoot position in a cavus foot, it is important to distinguish between an inverted calcaneus secondary to forefoot compensation and an uncompensated or partially compensated rearfoot varus. How is this done?**

A valgus wedge is placed under the lateral forefoot. If the heel everts to perpendicular, then the inverted rearfoot was secondary to forefoot compensation. If the heel remains inverted with the forefoot wedge, then the inverted rearfoot represents an uncompensated or partially compensated rearfoot varus. This can also be accomplished by having the patient with the forefoot off the edge of a step, thus eliminating the forefoot influence on the rearfoot. If the heel everts to perpendicular, then the inverted rearfoot was secondary to forefoot compensation. If the heel remains inverted, then the inverted rearfoot represents an uncompensated or partially compensated rearfoot varus.

○ **What surgical procedure addresses the frontal plane component of posterior cavus or rearfoot varus?**

The Dwyer calcaneal osteotomy, an extra-articular procedure addresses this component of cavus foot.

○ **Will the reduction of a fixed (rigid) anterior cavus deformity lead to significant reduction of the calcaneal inclination angle (posterior cavus)?**

Yes it will.

○ **Is a true ankle equinus (osseous, gastrocnemius, gastrosoleus) a common component of cavus foot?**

No! it is exceedingly <u>rare.</u> Inappropriate gastrocnemius or triceps surgery may produce severe complications, especially talipes calcaneus type of appropulsive gait.

○ **Do rigid hammertoes influence the evaluation of anterior cavus deformity?**

Yes. The reverse buckling influence of the digits must be released in order to evaluate the flexibility of the anterior cavus.

○ **Do radiographs help determine the rigidity or flexibility of anterior cavus?**

Yes. If significant reduction in the cavus deformity is noted on comparison of the weight bearing and non-weight bearing lateral radiographs, some degree of flexibility is assured.

○ **What is the role of plantar fasciotomies in cavus foot surgery?**

Fasciotomies are used to reduce the contracture of the plantar aponeurosis that is typical of a cavus foot. These releases are generally reserved for the adolescent or pediatric patient when only forefoot deformities are present.

○ **What is the difference between a subcutaneous plantar fasciotomy and a Steindler Stripping?**

A subcutaneous fasciotomy releases only the plantar aponeurosis. The Steindler stripping releases both the plantar aponeurosis and the plantar musculature.

○ **What are the effects of transferring the long extensor tendons to the metatarsal heads or to the midtarsus?**

It eliminates deforming forces on the digits .
It helps compensate for muscle imbalance responsible for creating flexible cavus.
It increases or maintains ankle dorsiflexory power.

○ **What is a Jones Suspension?**

An isolated transfer of the extensor hallucis longus to the neck of the first metatarsal. Additionally, the hallux IPJ is fused. This procedure compensates for an overpowering peroneus longus and flexor hallucis longus.

○ **What is a prerequisite for a Jones Suspension?**

An adequate dorsiflexory range of motion of the first ray.

○ **What are the consequences of over-correction following a Jones Suspension?**

Hallux limitus.

○ **What is a Heyman Procedure?**

Transfer of all five long extensor tendons to their respective metatarsal heads. This procedure helps to reduce flexible anterior cavus. This procedure is rarely used today. It is technically difficult and has many complications.

○ **What is the Hibbs Procedure?**

Transfer of the extensor digitorum longus to the third cuneiform to reduce a flexible anterior cavus. The original description included a plantar fascia and plantar muscle release.

○ **What is a STATT Procedure?**

The split tibialis anterior tendon transfer is an adjunctive procedure for treatment of flexible cavus foot. The lateral one half of the anterior tibial tendon is anastomosed to the peroneus tertius tendon near its insertion into the base of the fifth metatarsal. This is used when the EHL and EDL muscles are weak but the anterior tibial is a full strength.

○ **What is the purpose of the peroneus longus tendon transfer to the lesser tarsus?**

This transfer is used to help increase ankle dorsiflexion power and to reduce the drop foot component often seen with pes cavus. It also helps reduce plantarflexory force of the first ray.

○ **How is the peroneus longus tendon transfer done?**

The tendon is sectioned at the lateral cuboid, routed through the interosseous membrane, from lateral to anterior, and transferred down the EDL tendon sheath and inserted into the lesser tarsus.

○ **What is the purpose of the tibialis posterior tendon transfer?**

This transfer is used when weak anterior group muscles causes a dropfoot. This transfer may require rearfoot stabilization (fusion) due to loss of the major supinator of the foot.

○ **How is the tibialis posterior tendon transfer done?**

The tendon is sectioned at the navicular tuberosity, the tendon is routed through the interosseous membrane, from posterior to anterior, and transferred down the EDL tendon sheath and inserted into the lesser tarsus.

○ **What is the purpose of the peroneal anastomosis?**

This procedure decreases the plantarflexory force on the first ray and increases the eversion force of the foot. The procedure is used as an adjunctive procedure only.

○ **How is the peroneal anastomosis done?**

The peroneal longus is secured to the peroneus brevis at the level of the lateral ankle.

○ **What is a Cole Procedure?**

A lesser tarsal osteotomy designed to reduce a fixed anterior cavus. It preserves subtalar and midtarsal motion. It does not correct varus of the calcaneus or compensate for muscle imbalance.

○ **How is the Cole procedure done?**

This is a dorsal wedge osteotomy, apex plantarly, base dorsally, which extends from the cuboid laterally to opposite sides of the navicular-cuneiform joint medially. After the wedge is excised the forefoot is dorsiflexed to close the osteotomy and is fixated with pins or screws. A fasciotomy is performed if necessary to release a tight fascia.

○ **What are the disadvantages of the Cole procedure?**

This osteotomy results in a shorter, thicker, wider foot because the deformity is corrected by shortening of the dorsal convex surface of the foot.

○ **What is a Japas Procedure?**

This is a midtarsal "V" shaped osteotomy in which the apex is proximal, usually within the navicular, and the lateral limb of the "V" extends through the cuboid while the medial limb extends through the first cuneiform. The medial limb can extend through the first metatarsal base when a plantarflexed first metatarsal is present. No bone is excised. The proximal part of the distal bone segment is then shifted dorsally on the proximal segment elevating the forefoot and correcting the cavus. Pins are used to fixate the osteotomy. A fasciotomy is performed first.

○ **What are the disadvantages of the Cole and Japas procedures?**

Both procedures are difficult to control accurately and both cause significant trauma to the lesser tarsal - midtarsal area. Healing is slow and the amount of correction possible is less than with a triple arthrodesis. They generally result in less than a cosmetically pleasing result.

○ **What is the Truncated Tarsometatarsal Wedge Arthrodesis described by Jahss.**

This is the excision of a dorsal truncated wedge of bone across the tarsometatarsal joints. The degree of anterior cavus determines the amount of bone resected at each joint. Sagittal and frontal plane corrections are possible. The plantar fascia, which is not released, helps hold the forefoot in its corrected position. Internal fixation is said to be unnecessary. It is casted as usual.

O   What is the McElvenny-Caldwell procedure?

This is a first metatarsal cuneiform fusion for correction of a plantarflexed first metatarsal type of anterior cavus. It is useful in neuromuscular disease to provide stabilization.

O   Can a fixed anterior cavus be reduced by multiple dorsal wedge osteotomies of two or more metatarsals?

Yes.

O   What are the advantages of correcting fixed anterior cavus deformity at the metatarsal level?

This preserves the function of the major joints of the lesser tarsals and rearfoot. Differences in the level of individual metatarsals can be corrected at the time of surgery. Disability is less than with more proximal osteotomies. These procedures can easily be done in conjunction with muscle-tendon balancing procedures.

O   What is a Dwyer osteotomy?

This is a lateral closing wedge osteotomy of the calcaneus used to correct a rigid calcaneovarus deformity. The calcaneus must be unable to evert to the perpendicular when weight bearing with the forefoot influence eliminated.

O   What are the indications for the Dwyer osteotomy?

A rigid calcaneovarus deformity. The calcaneus must be unable to evert to the perpendicular when weight bearing with the forefoot influence eliminated.

O   How is the Dwyer osteotomy performed?

A laterally based wedge of bone is removed from the calcaneus just inferior and posterior to the peroneus longus tendon and parallel to it. The osteotomy is closed and fixated thus correcting the calcaneal varus. The complete correction of the varus must be obtained.

O   Describe the crescentic, biplane calcaneal osteotomy developed by Samilson.

This is a crescentic osteotomy at the posterior aspect of the calcaneus in which the posterior calcaneus is rotated dorsally, and any varus is derotated as well. This allows reduction of the calcaneal inclination angle or sagittal plane deformity as well as any frontal plane varus.

O   What is the danger of a dorsiflexory calcaneal osteotomy to correct posterior cavus?

As a result of raising the posterior calcaneus or reducing the calcaneal inclination angle, any rigid anterior cavus deformity present will cause the talus to rock into further dorsiflexion at the ankle joint. This will worsen pseudo equinus. This can be avoided by correcting any fixed anterior cavus simultaneously.

O   What are the two maneuvers which may be used during triple arthrodesis to effect correction at the midtarsal and subtalar joints?

Wedge resections.
Displacing or sliding maneuvers.

❍   **What is the order of joint resections during a triple arthrodesis?**

Midtarsal joint first, then subtalar joint.

❍   **What is the effect of posterior displacement of the calcaneus during triple arthrodesis?**

This increases the power of the posterior muscle group by increasing its lever arm at the ankle. The converse, anterior displacement of the calcaneus, is useful in spastic conditions when the posterior muscle group tends to overpower the anterior group.

COMMON REARFOOT PATHOLOGY AND SURGERY

○ **Name 3 systemic causes of heel pain.**

Gout, Rheumatoid arthritis, and seronegative arthropathy such as Reiter's syndrome and Ankylosing Spondylitis

○ **What is the Neutral Triangle of the calcaneus?**

The neutral triangle represents a radiolucent area seen on a lateral radiograph of the calcaneus. It is formed by pressure trabeculae from the subtalar joint combined with traction trabeculae formed by the normal pull of the Achilles tendon and plantar fascia.

○ **What is Forrester's disease?**

Diffuse idiopathic skeletal hyperostosis.

○ **Name 3 mechanical foot types associated with Haglund's deformity.**

Compensated rearfoot varus, compensated forefoot valgus, and rigid plantarflexed 1st ray.

○ **What is the normal value for the Fowler and Philip Angle?**

44-69 degrees.

○ **What is the Total Angle of Ruch?**

This is the combined value of the calcaneal inclination angle and the Fowler and Philip angle. A value of over 90 degrees is indicative of a Haglund's deformity.

○ **What are the borders of Kager's triangle?**

The superior calcaneal surface, the Achilles tendon and the long flexor tendons.

○ **Where is the retrocalcaneal synovial bursa located?**

This bursa separates the Achilles tendon from the superior 1/3 of the posterior surface of the calcaneus.

○ **Where is the adventitious superficial Achilles bursa located?**

This bursa is located between the Achilles tendon and the subcutaneous tissue.

○ **Under what circumstances is the Keck and Kelly procedure appropriate in the treatment of Haglund's deformity?**

When there is a structural cavus foot with a high calcaneal inclination angle but a normal postero-superior prominence that is symptomatic.

❍   **What is Heel Spur Syndrome?**

The symptom complex of plantar stress, tendinitis, fasciitis, with or without the presence of an inferior calcaneal spur.

❍   **Which nerve is often implicated as a cause of inferior calcaneal pain?**

The nerve to the abductor digiti quinti muscle, referred to as Baxter's nerve, is commonly believed to be a source of heel pain.

❍   **What is the DuVries incisional approach for heel spur surgery?**

Medial horizontal approach.

❍   **What are the advantages of using a plantar approach for heel spur surgery?**

Direct visualization of exostosis, avoidance of medial calcaneal nerve branches, easy access to the subcalcaneal adventitious bursa.

❍   **Where does the subcalcaneal adventitious bursa form?**

Between the most prominent point of the tuberosity and the plantar fat pad.

❍   **What are the differential diagnoses for heel spur syndrome?**

Plantar fasciitis, subcalcaneal adventitious bursitis, policeman's heel (contusion, stone bruise), tendinitis of intrinsic muscles, nerve entrapment, heel neuroma, herniation of plantar fascia, painful piezogenic papules, radiculopathy, infection, and systemic disease.

❍   **What is the primary structure that supplies venous drainage to the heel?**

Small saphenous vein.

❍   **What are the differential diagnoses of posterior heel pain?**

Haglund's deformity, retrocalcaneal bursitis, Achilles tendinitis, calcifications within the Achilles tendon, systemic arthritides, DISH.

❍   **What are the incisional approaches for Haglund's deformity?**

Fowler and Philip direct posterior, lateral linear, lateral lazy L, 2 incisional.

❍   **What does "chasing the bump" refer to in Haglund's deformity surgery?**

This refers to the excessive resection of the posterior-superior prominence and compromise of the insertion of the Achilles tendon by successively resecting the bony prominence created by the previous use of the osteotome for bony removal.

❍   **What is the Miller and Vogel procedure?**

A surgical procedure used for Haglund's deformity, which combines the Keck and Kelly procedure with resection of the posterior-superior prominence and using internal fixation.

○ **Where does the calcaneus receive its blood supply?**

Via calcaneal branches of the posterior tibial artery and lateral plantar artery medially, by communicating branches of the peroneal and lateral malleolar arteries laterally and communicating branches posteriorly.

○ **What cystic lesion of bone is commonly seen in the calcaneus?**

Unicameral bone cyst.

○ **What are the three types of tarsal coalitions?**

Syndesmosis (fibrous), synchondrosis (cartilaginous), and synostosis (bony).

○ **Which tarsal coalition has the highest prevalence?**

Middle facet STJ coalition.

○ **Which radiographic view is best used to visualize a Calcaneo-Navicular coalition?**

High angle medial oblique.

○ **What are the three branches of the posterior tibial nerve?**

Medial plantar, lateral plantar, and medial calcaneal nerves.

○ **What are the advantages of endoscopic plantar fasciotomy in the surgical treatment of heel spur surgery?**

Decreased levels of soft tissue damage and postoperative pain.

○ **What is the postoperative care for endoscopic plantar fasciotomy?**

Immediate full weightbearing, but avoid excessive ambulation. Patient returns to regular shoes with orthotic devices as soon as tolerated.

○ **What is the "Windlass action" of the plantar fascia?**

This is the action that raises the longitudinal arch as the metatarsophalangeal joints are dorsiflexed and the plantar fascia tightens.

○ **How does a calcaneal stress fracture appear radiographically?**

Lateral radiograph: vertical sclerotic band with the normal trabecular pattern running perpendicular to the line of the stress fracture.

○ **With a stress fracture of the calcaneus, when do routine radiographs become positive?**

Within 3-4 weeks following the onset of symptoms.

○ **Name 4 conservative methods of treating heel pain syndrome?**

Rest, NSAIDs, steroid injections, and iontophoresis.

O   **What is the postoperative course for a plantar fasciotomy via a plantar incision?**

Nonweightbearing 3 wks, then patient is changed to a postoperative shoe for several more weeks.

O   **How is Superficial Achilles Bursitis treated?**

Shoe modification, heel lift, softening of the heel counter of the shoe.

O   **What is a Kidner procedure?**

Excision of an accessory navicular with advancement of the posterior tibial tendon plantarly.

O   **When excising an accessory navicular or hypertrophic navicular tuberosity, how much bone should be resected?**

The hypertrophic tuberosity should be resected flush with the medial cuneiform.

O   **What are the indications for a Kidner procedure?**

The Kidner procedure is not a corrective procedure for flatfoot deformity; it should be used for symptomatic prominence about an enlarged navicular tuberosity.

O   **What anatomical structures must be encountered when excising an accessory navicular bone?**

Communicating branches of the greater saphenous vein (medial marginal vein), saphenous nerve, and posterior tibial tendon.

O   **What is the postoperative course status post Kidner procedure?**

NWB BK cast with foot in equinovarus x 4wks, then BK partially WB cast with well molded arch X 4 wks, then full WB with firm orthosis.

O   **Name 3 accessory ossicles of the rearfoot and their corresponding anatomic locations.**

Os trigonum- posterior talus; Os tibiale externum-navicular tuberosity; Os peroneum- cuboid.

O   **What venous structures must be encountered when performing soft tissue dissection along the navicular tuberosity?**

Medial marginal vein system.

O   **What radiographic view is helpful when evaluating for tarsal coalition (STJ)?**

Harris-Beath view.

O   **When resecting a symptomatic os trigonum, which tendinous structure must be retracted carefully and not transected?**

Flexor Hallucis Longus.

O   **Which ligament must be transected when performing a tarsal tunnel release?**

Laciniate ligament (flexor retinaculum).

○ **Which is the last rearfoot bone to appear radiographically after birth?**

Navicular.

○ **Where does the medial aspect of the heel receive its circulation?**

Calcaneal branches of posterior tibial and lateral plantar arteries.

○ **What is the most common complication seen after total plantar fasciotomy?**

Lateral column pain (cuboid syndrome).

○ **What is the only rearfoot bone with no tendinous attachments?**

Talus.

○ **What foot types are commonly seen in patients presenting with Haglund's deformity?**

Compensated rearfoot varus, compensated forefoot valgus, rigid plantarflexed 1st ray.

○ **At what age does the calcaneal apophysis typically close?**

14-16 years of age.

○ **How would a calcaneal stress fracture appear on bone scan (Triphasic technetium)?**

Increased uptake in all 3 phases.

○ **What is the mechanism typically involved in anterior process fractures of the calcaneus?**

Plantarflexion on a supinated foot.

○ **What is the clinical presentation of a patient with "os trigonum syndrome?"**

Generalized rearfoot pain or aching, pain may be more posterior lateral, increases with activity, decreases with rest, pain may be exacerbated with motion of hallux, pain may be exacerbated with ankle plantarflexion, palpation deep behind lateral malleolus elicit pain, may see posterior lateral edema.

○ **What is a saddle bone deformity?**

A metatarsal cuneiform exostosis.

○ **Neuritis of what nerve is sometimes associated with a saddle bone deformity?**

Deep peroneal nerve.

○ **What is an in-step plantar fasciotomy?**

This is a fasciotomy performed on the plantar aspect of the foot, anterior to the heel, over the medial band of the plantar fascia. It is performed through a small transverse or linear incision. The superficial fatty tissue is separated allowing visualization of the fascia which is gently incised while the forefoot is gently dorsiflexed.

○ **What is ESWT (Extracorporeal Shock Wave Therapy)?**

Extracorporeal Shock Wave Therapy (ESWT) is a procedure used to treat chronic heel pain ie. Plantar fasciitis. This is a non-invasive surgical procedure in which strong sound waves are directed at the area of the heel which is painful and induce a healing response by the body.

DERMATOLOGY

○ **How many layers are there in the epidermis?**

The four layers of the epidermis are:
>   the stratum corneum or outermost layer
>   the stratum lucidum (clear cell layer) (only seen on palms and soles)
>   the stratum granulosum
>   the stratum spinosum (stratum malpighii)(spiny/prickle cell) layer
>   the stratum germinativum or cuboidal or columnar stratum basale (basal layer) on the basement
membrane.

○ **What are the tissue layers of the skin?**

The epidermis, dermis and subcutaneous layers.

○ **What is a macule?**

A macule is a primary skin lesion that is circumscribed alteration in the color of the skin, not visibly raised or depressed, or presenting any change in the consistency of the skin; examples are freckles or tattoo marks.

○ **What is a patch?**

A patch is a primary skin lesion that is a larger macule. It is greater than 1cm in diameter.

○ **What is a papule?**

A papule is a primary lesion. It is a small elevation above the skin level varying in size from 1mm to 1 cm in diameter. An example would be a small elevated nevus or wart.

○ **What is a plaque?**

A plaque is primary lesion that is elevated above the skin level and greater than 1cm in diameter. An example could be a > 1 cm corn or wart.

○ **What is a nodule?**

A nodule is a primary lesion that is solid and larger than 1cm in diameter consisting of inflammatory cellular infiltrates or neoplasm.

○ **What is a wheal?**

A wheal is a primary lesion which is a plateau-like elevation produced by edema in the upper corium and the leaking of blood plasma through the vessels walls. Mosquito bites start as wheals.

○ **What is a vesicle?**

A vesicle is primary lesion that is a circumscribed elevation of the skin measuring less than 5 mm in diameter and is fluid filled. An example would be a lesion of herpes simplex or acute tinea pedis.

○ **What is a bulla?**

A bulla is a primary lesion that is larger than 5 mm and produced by factors such as chemicals, heat and friction (friction blister), as well as primary skin conditions such as bullous pemphigoid. Some require that blisters be ≤1 cm before using the term bullae.

○ **What is a pustule?**

A pustule is a primary skin lesion that is a circumscribed liquid accumulation of free pus as seen in acne or impetigo.

○ **What is a skin tumor?**

A tumor is a primary lesion of new growth, varying size and composed of skin and subcutaneous tissue. It can be either benign or malignant.

○ **What are secondary lesions?**

Secondary lesions evolve over time from primary lesions usually because of scratching or infection.

○ **What is a scale?**

A scale is a secondary skin lesion. It is exfoliation of accumulated debris of dead stratum corneum and results from imperfect cornification; examples are scales of psoriasis, tinea and dandruff.

○ **What is a crust?**

A crust is a secondary skin lesion. It is a coagulation product of blood, serum, pus or a combination of two or more of these. Examples are scabs of impetigo.

○ **What is an excoriation?**

An excoriation is secondary lesion that represents a superficial loss of epidermis as a result of scratching or rubbing.

○ **What is a fissure?**

A fissure is a secondary change in the skin that presents as a linear superficial crack in the epidermis. Often seen within hyperkeratotic heel rims.

○ **What is an erosion?**

An erosion is a secondary lesion. It is a shallow scooped-out superficial loss of all or part of the epidermis. Often seen in interdigital tinea pedis.

○ **What is an ulcer?**

An ulcer is a secondary skin lesion. It is damaged skin of varying depth. A result of a destructive process of the epidermis that may extend deep to the dermis, subcutis or even bone.

○ **How are Stage one (National Pressure Ulcer Classification) pressure ulcers be staged and treated?**

Stage one pressure ulcers appear as non-blanchable erythema of intact skin, the heralding lesion of skin ulceration. Often seen over a bony prominence from prolonged pressure or shoe irritation. Discoloration of the skin, warmth edema, induration, hyperkeratosis or hardness may also be indicators. Paring of hyperkeratosis and/or pressure relief are appropriate management measures.

○ **How are stage two (National Pressure Ulcer Classification) pressure ulcers be staged and treated?**

Stage two pressure ulcers have partial-thickness skin loss involving epidermis, dermis or both. The ulcer is superficial and presents clinically as an abrasion, blister or shallow crater. Pressure relief, topical antibiotic and simple dressing are indicated.

○ **How are stage three (National Pressure Ulcer Classification) pressure ulcers be staged and treated?**

Stage three pressure ulcers represent full-thickness skin loss involving damage to, or necrosis of the subcutaneous tissue that may extend down to but not through the underlying fascia. The ulcer presents clinically as a deep crater with or without undermining of adjacent tissue. Vascular workup, systemic antibiosis, pressure relief and wound care should be considered.

○ **How are stage four (National Pressure Ulcer Classification) pressure ulcers staged and treated?**

Stage four pressure ulcers represent full-thickness skin loss with extensive destruction, tissue necrosis, or damage to muscle, bone, tendon, joint capsule. Undermining and sinus tracts also may be associated with Stage Four pressure ulcers. Hospitalization for vascular workup, operative surgical debridement, systemic antibiosis and wound care should be considered.

○ **How is a keloid defined?**

Keloid is aggressive scar tissue that extends beyond the area of original trauma.

○ **What is lichenification?**

Lichenification is thickening of the skin with exaggeration of the normal skin lines. Hyperpigmentation scaling and pruritus often accompany. Favors anterior ankles and suggests repetitive rubbing or scratching.

○ **What are telangiectasias?**

Telangiectasia are visible dilated superficial blood vessels seen in connection with certain heritable diseases, e.g. familial telangiectasia; associated with liver diseases and pregnancy and as a sequel to x-ray treatment. Often seen about the ankles in the elderly.

○ **How is a KOH examination performed?**

Scrape epidermal flakes to glass slide, apply 20% KOH, warm or use dimethyl sulfoxide solvent (DMSO), wait ten minutes, examine under low power and reduced light.

○ **What is the diagnostic finding on a KOH examination in chronic tinea pedis?**

Segmented branching hyphae.

○ **What are Koen's tumors?**

Multiple firm periungual fibromas associated with tuberous sclerosis.

○ **Describe the clinical findings in epidermolysis bullosa (EB) simplex.**

EB presents as spontaneous blisters of the fingers toes knees or elbows from minor trauma beginning at birth or early childhood. The blisters heal without scarring. The disease is due to defects in keratins 5 and 14 and is an autosomal dominant trait.

❍ **What is a papulosquamous skin disorder?**

Any of a number of erythematous or purple papules and plaques topped with scales.

❍ **Which papulosquamous diseases can be seen on the foot or ankle?**

Psoriasis, lichen planus, lichen nitidus and pityriasis rubra pilaris can be seen on the foot and ankle.

❍ **Describe the characteristic rash of pityriasis rosea.**

Pink to erythematous maculo-papular rash of the chest and or back following a viral infection. Spares the soles. Starting with a single 2-4 cm sharply defined thin oval plaques with a characteristic collarette of scale then within a few days to weeks, crops of similar but smaller lesions follow and resolve spontaneously.

❍ **What is pompholyx?**

Pompholyx is an episodic vesiculobullous eczema of the palms and soles especially edges of fingers. Multiple deep-seated pruritic nits and evolving vesicles.

❍ **What is an id reaction and how is it managed?**

Immune mediated, sympathetic response to acute tinea. Sterile eruptions distant from the acute site i.e.: fingers palms chest or back. Treat the primary tinea and the id reaction will resolve with it.

❍ **Explain the pathogenesis of allergic contact dermatitis.**

Allergic contact dermatitis is a delayed cell mediated hypersensitivity reaction. First a hapten contacts skin and forms a protein complex. Langerhans skin cell present the complete antigen to the T-helper cell causing mediator release. Sensitization takes 5-21 days. Upon re-exposure there is proliferation of activated T cells, mediator release and migration of cytotoxic T cells resulting in cutaneous eczematous inflammation at the site of contact. This takes 4-72 hours after re-exposure. Small exposure can trigger eruptions in sensitized persons.

❍ **Name the two types of contact dermatitis.**

Primary irritant and allergic contact dermatitis.

❍ **How is patch testing done?**

Patch testing is necessary to distinguish between irritant contact dermatitis and allergic dermatitis. A small amount of allergen in a petrolatum base is applied in individual aluminum wells affixed to a strip of paper tape applied to the patient's upper back for 48 hours and read for erythema edema and vesiculation then and again at 72 and 96 hours for delayed reactions indicative of allergic reaction.

❍ **How is contact dermatitis managed?**

Identify and remove allergen. Protection measures. Cool compresses and topical steroids.

❍ **How are the bullous diseases classified/defined?**

Bullous diseases are classified by the depth of involvement, either within the epidermis or below the epidermis.

❍ **What are several intra-epidermal bullous diseases?**

Allergic contact dermatitis, epidermal bullosa simplex, bullous diabeticorum, herpes simplex and zoster are all examples of intra-epidermal bullous diseases.

❍ **What are several sub-epidermal bullous diseases?**

Bullous pemphigoid, dystrophic epidermal bullosa and porphyria cutanea tarda are a few examples of sub-epidermal bullous diseases.

❍ **What special tests may be necessary to diagnose blistering diseases of the skin?**

Cultures for bacteria, smears for viruses, biopsy with direct immunofluorescence are all helpful in diagnosing skin disease.

❍ **What are some drugs that can cause vesiculobullous eruptions?**

Tetracycline, sulfonamides, vancomycin, lithium, thiazides, furosemide, and naproxen all can cause vesiculobullous eruptions.

❍ **What are the more common pustular skin eruptions?**

Folliculitis, impetigo and acne.

❍ **What do the lesions of pustular psoriasis contain?**

Only leukocytes, no bacteria.

❍ **Describe the characteristic primary lesion of lichen planus.**

Pruritic purple and pink papules and plaques on the flexor wrists. Pterygium nail dystrophy may occur.

❍ **What are the characteristic oral findings in lichen planus?**

Wickham's striae, a white netlike or reticulated, patterned discoloration of the buccal mucosa.

❍ **Describe the isomorphic response in lichen planus?**

The development of new lesions in response to external trauma or scratching.

❍ **What is lichen simplex chronicus?**

A perpetuating itch scratch cycle creating chronic often lichenified plaque.

❍ **How is lichen simplex chronicus treated?**

Stop scratching and frictional trauma. Often responds to occlusive topical steroid therapy.

❍ **How does granuloma annulare usually present clinically?**

Typically presents with violaceous or flesh-colored dermal papules arranged in an annular configuration affecting dorsum of hands and feet.

O   **What is the usual clinical course of granuloma annulare?**

Classic granuloma annulare spontaneous resolves but can recur.

O   **How do adverse drug reactions differ from true drug allergies?**

True drug allergies are immune mediated.

O   **What are some typical cutaneous reactions to drugs?**

Pruritus, erythema, macular to papular eruptions, urticaria, angioedema, erythema multiforme and exfoliative dermatitis.

O   **Which drugs commonly cause photo eruptions?**

Drugs causing photo eruptions include sulfonamides, thiazides, oral hypoglycemics NSAIDs and griseofulvin.

O   **What is vasculitis?**

Inflammation of blood vessels.

O   **What is leukocytoclastic vasculitis?**

Purpuric papules most often on the extremities associated with many immune mediated diseases, infections, drugs, or malignancy. Also know as palpable purpura or necrotizing vasculitis.

O   **List several key features of Henoch-Schönlein purpura (HSP).**

Intermittent purpura of the extremities and buttocks usually affecting children. Abdominal pain, arthralgia and hematuria may accompany the purpura.

O   **List three diseases that a Wood's lamp can be used as an aide in diagnosis?**

Erythrasma, tinea capitis, tinea versicolor. Tinea pedis does not glow.

O   **What the primary lesions of vitiligo?**

Hypopigmented patches and macules.

O   **List the clinical features of tuberous sclerosis?**

Multiple sebaceous adenoma, mental retardation and Koen's tumors.

O   **What cutaneous lesions are seen with Hansen's disease?**

Cutaneous numbness, neutrophic ulcers, erythema nodosum, and erythematous macules and eyebrow loss.

O   **What is erythema nodosum?**

Inflammatory nodules and infiltrates in the subcutaneous layers of the lower extremities associated with a Streptococcus infection, sarcoidosis or drugs especially oral contraceptives.

O   **What causes acne?**

Heredity, androgens, abnormal keratinization and Propionibacterium acnes all play a roll in acne.

○   **What is hidradenitis suppurativa?**

This is a chronic recurrent axillary or groin deep skin infections of the apocrine glands. Abscesses and sinus tracts often develop.

○   **What is rosacca?**

Rosacea presents with telangiectasia, sebaceous gland hyperplasia and acne of the forehead cheeks nose and chin in the elderly. Mite infestation might play a role.

○   **What are the key skin features of lupus erythematosus?**

Malar erythematous facial rash and psoriasiform eruptions in a photo exposed skin pattern.

○   **What are the key skin features of scleroderma?**

Scleroderma presents with morphea (firm sclerotic indurated plaques). The lesions are often multiple smooth topped with a white center and purple border.

○   **Which viruses cause acral-located lesions of the hands and or feet?**

Human papilloma virus, herpes simplex, herpes zoster and Coxsackie virus can be found on the hands or feet.

○   **What is porokeratosis plantaris discreta?**

PPD is a small plantar focal hyperkeratosis with a central horny plug that is probably a pressure induced keratosis. Some believe it is a plugged eccrine duct or cyst.

○   **What is the appropriate surgical anatomical inferior boundary when curetting plantar warts?**

The dense superficial fascia of the sole is the boundary, not the basement membrane histological feature.

○   **Which organism usually causes chronic tinea pedis?**

Usually Trichophyton rubrum causes the dry form of tinea pedis.

○   **Which organism usually causes vesicular tinea pedis?**

Usually Trichophyton mentagrophytes causes the blistering form of tinea pedis.

○   **How can chronic tinea pedis that has been resistant to topical therapies be treated?**

Oral terbinafine 250mg qd for two weeks or itraconazole 400 mg qd for one week can be tried.

○   **Which clinical types of onychomycosis are associated with AIDS?**

Both white superficial and proximal subungual onychomycosis have been associated with AIDS.

○   **Which fungal organism causes more than 90% of onychomycosis?**

Trichophyton rubrum.

❍   **What are the most effective FDA approved oral treatment regimes for pedal onychomycosis?**

Itraconazole 200mg qd for three months and terbinafine 250mg qd for three months.

❍   **What causes juvenile plantar dermatosis or "wet foot dry foot" syndrome?**

Hyperhidrosis that dries out too quickly when occlusive footgear is removed in dry air.

❍   **What is effective prevention for juvenile plantar dermatosis or "wet foot dry foot" syndrome?**

Prompt application of emollients like A& D ointment or Vaseline each time shoes are removed.

❍   **A pigmented lesion's width is suspicious when its diameter reaches what dimension?**

Melanoma should be suspected when a pigmented lesions grows larger 6 mm or the diameter of a pencil eraser.

❍   **Which different anatomical surfaces are affected by psoriasis and lichen planus?**

Generally psoriasis affects extensor surfaces and lichen planus affects flexor surfaces and mucous membranes.

❍   **What is the chief diagnostic histological feature seen in plantar verrucae?**

Basilar intracellular inclusion bodies.

❍   **What is the chief diagnostic histological feature seen in porokeratosis plantaris discreta?**

Hyperkeratosis and coronoid lamellae formation.

❍   **What histological feature distinguishes pressure induced hyperkeratosis from inherited hyperkeratosis (keratoderma).**

The stratum granulosum cell layer is maintained in inherited keratodermas while it is lost in the central highest pressure areas of pressure keratoses.

❍   **What are the key features of treating plantar psoriasis?**

Tars, tretinoin, pulsed high potency topical corticosteroids under occlusion coupled with calcipotriene (Dovonex≤) have all shown usefulness in plantar psoriasis.

❍   **What causes pitted keratolysis?**

Hyperhidrosis with overgrowth of Micrococcus sedentarius causes the superficial erosive horny pits.

❍   **How does one manage pedal scabies?**

Topical permethrin (Elimite), sulphur or chlordane (Lindane≤) applied ear to toes have all been used to clear pedal scabies.

DIABETES MELLITUS

○ **What are the three forces that cause ulcerations in the foot?**

Friction: is the resistance that any body meets in moving over another body, the more irregular the surfaces in contact, the greater the increase in friction. So the more irregular the shape of the foot, the greater the risk of friction induced tissue breakdown.

Pressure: is the force of one body onto another, by its weight. For a given wt, the pressure is inversely proportional to the area the foot rests on. So increase the area and decrease the pressure.

Shear Force: is the combination of frictional and compressive forces. This is believed to be the force most responsible for tissue breakdown in the insensitive foot.

○ **What are the classifications used in evaluating ulcerations of the foot?**

Wagner's - was one of the original classifications and still the most widely used.
　Grade 0 - Skin is intact, but there may be some osseous deformity.
　Grade 1 - Localized superficial ulcer.
　Grade 2 - Deep ulcer with extension to tendon, bone, ligament, or joint.
　Grade 3 - Deep abscess with osteomyelitis.
　Grade 4 - Gangrene of the toes or forefoot.
　Grade 5 - Gangrene of the whole foot.

The University of Texas Diabetic Foot Classification System: This is a newer based system similar to Wagner's with a couple of additional risk factors added. The system relies on three questions - how deep is the ulcer?, is it ischemic?, and is the wound infected?

○ **What are the risk factors for diabetic foot ulceration?**

Peripheral Neuropathy which is probably the most significant single risk factor.
Deformity & Decreased Joint Motility usually increases the shear force to which the foot is subjected.
Poor Glucose Control increases the patient risk to neuropathy, decreased wound healing, PVD, and decreased immune function.
History of Previous Ulceration & Amputation will cause plantar pressure distribution to be changed, therefore increasing the risk of amputation.
*As you increase the number of risk factors the patient develops, you increase the risk that the patient will develop an ulcer, so they are cumulative.

○ **What are the various treatments for foot ulceration?**

Decrease the Pressure: This can be done by a variety of methods.

Felted foam dressings: A piece of felted foam is cut out to accommodate the ulcer and is applied to the foot via rubber cement and is changed once a week.

Total contact cast: This is a cast made to decrease the amount of force the foot is subject to, by increasing the total surface area.

Accommodative Orthotics: These are very important once the ulcer is healed to reduce the risk of recurrence.

Surgery: Excision of a bony prominence, possible plastic surgery i.e. skin flap

Growth factors & Skin substitutes: These have not yet been proven to be as effective as the above but could be good adjunctive therapy. The single most effective treatment for foot ulcerations is bed rest! Blood Supply: If the patient does not have good perfusion to the foot then the ulcer will never heal, the patient might only need a vascular by-pass, or to increase there cardiac output.

Glucose Control: Poor glucose control affects the immune system (decreases white cell function), and decreases the soft tissue cross linking through production of advanced glycosylation products.

Dressings: 1/4 strength Betadine≤ BID, or NS wet to dry BID, hydrogel, and Aquagel≤ can be used also.

○   **What are the qualities of the diabetic foot that makes it different from the norm?**

Decreased vibratory, pinprick, and light tough.
Muscle atrophy and weakness (intrinsic muscle wasting).
Patients develop cocked-up toes, plantar prominent met heads, equinus deformity, varus deformity of the hindfoot.
Decreased DTR's of the patella and Achilles.
*All these things decrease the ability of the foot to compensate for irregularities of terrain, and increase the risk for ulceration.

○   **What are the findings in the neuropathic foot?**

Well nourished tissue.
Good dorsalis pedis & posterior tibial pulses.
Decreased or absent sensation, vibration sense, and Achilles tendon reflex.
Tendency for hammer toes and high foot arch.
Calluses at pressure points.
Charcot deformities.
Foot drop.
Superimposed infections: ulcers, osteomyelitis.
Paresthesia, hyperesthesia, hypoesthesia, and radicular pain.
Anhydrosis.

○   **What causes the patient to develop a neuropathic foot?**

There are two schools of thought: Vascular basis vs Hyperglycemia. Up to now the evidence suggest that the symmetric neuropathy can develop in the absence of a clear-cut vascular or hypoxia basis and it likely results from a metabolic defect whereas the focal lesions may have a vascular basis.

Hyperglycemia causes increased activity of the polyol pathway in nerves that fluctuates
with the level of plasma glucose, hyperglycemia causes increased levels of glucose, sorbitol, and fructose in the nerve, and these levels rapidly reduce to normal when insulin is introduced. Hyperglycemia > Increased nerve glucose > increased polyol pathway activity > Decreased myo-inositol concentrations > Restriction on phosphatidylinositol turnover > decreased Na-K-ATPase activity > decreased NCV.

○   **What are the radiographic features of the neuropathic foot?**

Demineralization.
Osteolysis.
Charcot's joint.

○   **Name some other causes of peripheral neuropathy.**

Alcoholism, Herniated nucleus pulposus, Heavy metals, Vitamin deficiencies, Collagen diseases, Pernicious anemia, Malignancy, Pressure neuropathy, Uremia, Porphyria, Hansen's disease, and drugs.

○   **What are the various treatments for neuropathy?**

Hyperglycemia Control: Strict control of blood glucose levels can increase NCV. It was also shown that patients with elevated blood sugars had decreased pain threshold. Patients with poor glycemic control have quicker onset and more severe peripheral neuropathy.
Sorbinil: long acting aldose reductase inhibitor that slightly increases NCV.

○   **What is the treatment for painful neuropathy?**

First is strict glycemic control.
Second acetaminophen or ibuprofen, narcotics should be avoided due to the risk of abus since painful neuropathy can be chronic in nature.
Anticonvulsants have proven to be ineffective in chronic pain but may be of benefit in lancinating and paroxysmal pain.
Tricyclic antidepressants have proven beneficial in patients with depression combined with painful neuropathy.
Topical capsaicin cream is good for mild pain.
The newest agent Neurontin≤ has shown some promising results.

○   **What are the methods of diagnosis of diabetic peripheral neuropathy?**

Weinstein-Semmes monofilaments: loss of protective sensation occurs when the patient cannot feel a 10g filament.
Vibratory sensation: use a 256htz at the MPJ, midfoot, ankle, and tibial tubercle.
Pressure-Specified Sensory Device: the lowest threshold at which patients developed ulcers was, for one point static 9.1g/mm2, and two-point static threshold 32.9g/mm2.

○   **What are some of the atypical symptoms seen in a diabetic having a MI?**

Confusion, dyspnea, fatigue, and N/V can be the presenting symptoms in 42% of the population, whereas in the non-diabetic it is only 6-12%

○   **What are the risk factors for CAD in the diabetic?**

Asymptomatic Hyperglycemia: this is an independent risk factor for CAD, it has never been proven that tight blood glucose level control decrease the risk of CAD.
Lipid abnormalities: diabetics usually have a increased VLDL compared to the normal population and decreased LDL, and diabetics usually develop CAD at lower levels of LDL/VLDL.
Hyperinsulinemia: causes atherogenesis, low HDL levels, and hypertension.

○   **What is the treatment for Lactic Acidosis?**

It is focused on the correction of the pH; the patient should be given intravenous bicarbonate to maintain the plasma bicarbonate at 8 to 10 mmol/L and the pH above 7.1

○   **What is the treatment for diabetic ketoacidosis?**

Insulin: given 25 to 50 unit bolus I.V., then give 8 to 10 units/hr until the ketoacidosis is reversed.
Fluids: 1-2L of isotonic saline or LR rapidly IV, then should be determined by urine output.
If plasma glucose below 17 mmol/L then add 5% glucose solution to decrease risk of cerebral edema.
Potassium: as needed 3-4 hours after start of treatment.

Bicarbonate: only needed if pH<7.0, or if patient is hypotensive.

O   What are the complications seen in diabetic ketoacidosis?

Erosive gastritis, cerebral edema, hyperkalemia, hypoglycemia, hypokalemia, MI, mucormycosis, RDS, vascular thrombosis.

O   What are the signs and symptoms seen in Diabetic Ketoacidosis?

Anorexia, N/V, increased urine formation, abdominal pain, coma or mental stares changes, Kussmaul respirations, leukocytosis, labs: >K+, <MG++, <Na+, hypertriglyceridemia.

O   Diabetic nephropathy is clinically defined as?

By the presence of persistent proteinuria (.5g/24HR) in a patient with diabetes and concomitant retinopathy and elevated blood pressure.

O   What is the treatment of diabetic nephropathy?

Blood pressure control: delays the progression of diabetic nephropathy and retard the onset of overt renal disease.
Dietary Treatment: diet restricted to .5 to .6 g of protein/kg of body weight per day.
Glycemic Control: It is important to have tight glycemic control in the early stages of the syndrome, and it is less effective at the late stages.
Aldose Reductase.
Angiotensin II medications.

O   You have a 45 yr old NIDDM F with ESRD and a foot infection that has grown out MRSA and you want to put the patient on Vancomycin. You order a chem 7 and CBC: NA 140, K 4.5, Cl 101, CO₂ 29, Bun 38, Cr 3.5, WBC 12.7, Hgb 10.9, Hct 29.9, Plt 150. Pt wt is 59kg. What dose of Vancomycin would you give this patient?

First you must find the patient's Creatinine Clearance, so you need to use the formula Clcr(ml/min)= (140-age) X wt(kg)/72 X serum Cr (mg/dl)X.85 (for women), this pt Clcr is 22ml/mg which is decreased, so the patient would be started on 500mg q24-48hr; and then dosed according to the trough level.

O   Your patient is in the hospital for minor cellulitis and a draining 1st met ulcer, and you're having trouble controlling his glucose level. What are the possible causes of insulin resistance other then the infection?

Inflammation, MI or ischemia, Trauma, Sx, Emotional stress, Pregnancy, Glucocorticoid, Estrogens (birth control included), Sympathomimetic, Nicotinic acid, Antibodies to insulin, Antibodies to insulin receptors.

O   What are the autonomic manifestations seen in diabetes?

Cardiovascular: increased heart rate, orthostatic hypotension, decreased cardiac output; 20-40% of diabetics are affected.
Urogenital: Hesitancy, poor stream, feeling of inadequate bladder emptying, and incontinence, and these increase the risk for UTI and possibly accelerate end stage renal disease (ESRD).
GI: It effects the motility, secretions, and absorption, nausea, postprandial vomiting, bloating, loss of appetite. One study showed up to 76% of diabetics had some type of GI problems.
Sweating abnormalities.
Neuroglycopenia and Hypoglycemic Unawareness.

O   What factors in the diabetic could impede the healing of an ulceration?

Ischemia.
Poor glycemic control.
Callus formation over the ulcer.
Infection.
Malnutrition.
Peripheral neuropathy.
ESRD.
Cardiac abnormalities.
Poor wound care.
Patient non-compliance.
Bony prominence.

O **What are the signs of ischemic vascular disease?**

Dyshidrosis.
Atrophy of soft tissue.
Absence of hair.
Tendency to develop fissures on heels and prominences.
Diminished or absent DP/PT pulses.
Prolonged venous filling time (over 20 sec).
Rubor of toes or foot on dependency.
Blanching of foot on elevation.
Ankle/Arm index of less then .45mm/hg.

O **What are the two types of vascular disease the diabetic suffers from and where do they usually present in the lower extremity?**

Macroangiopathy: Is most often seen in popliteal and tibial arteries, Strand et al. found that 81% of diabetic patients have stenosis or occlusion of the three major vessels below the knee as compared with 57% of the normal population.

Microangiopathy: According to Cecile et al., 40 % of diabetics have characteristic lesions in the small arteries of the foot(arterioles and capillaries) and this usually precedes the large vessel disease.

O **You have a 38 yr old male going for surgery tomorrow with local and MAC and the patient must be NPO overnight. His insulin regimen is 25 units NPH A.M. and 20 units NPH P.M., he gets 8 units Reg. A.M. What would his insulin dose be in the morning and what fluids would you put him on? If he were on an oral agent, how would that change your management?**

The patient should get half his normal NPH dose in the A.M., and you would hold his regular insulin to decrease the risk of hypoglycemia. The patient should be started on 1/2D5W&NS at 60cc an hour at 6A.M. If the patient were on a oral agent then the drug should be held.

O **Briefly explain the Somogyi effect & the Dawn phenomenon.**

Somogyi Effect is a rebound hyperglycemia following an episode of hypoglycemia due to counter regulatory hormone release. The insulin dose should be decreased, this effect is more common in children.

Dawn phenomenon is an early rise in the morning plasma glucose that requires increased amounts of insulin to maintain euglycemia and is independent of the Somogyi effect. It is believed to be caused by the nocturnal surge of growth hormone release, to establish the difference between the two, a glucose check should be done at 3 am, since the two have very different Tx.

O **Briefly explain the symptoms of hypoglycemia and it's treatment.**

Symptoms

-Excessive secretion of epinephrine: sweating, tremor, tachycardia, anxiety, and hunger.

-CNS: dizziness, headache, clouding of vision, blunted mental acuity, lose of fine motor skills, confusion, abnormal behavior, convulsions, coma.

Treatment

-For serious episode: IV bolus of 25 to 50g glucose as a 50% solution followed by constant infusion of glucose until the patient can eat. Hypoglycemia from sulfonylureas may last for days and it is common for patients to lapse back into coma if glucose infusions are stopped to soon.

OSTEOMYELITIS IN DISEASES

○ **What is osteomyelitis?**

Nelaton is thought to be the first one to use the term osteomyelitis to describe an infection of bone and marrow in 1844. Infection of the cortex alone without marrow involvement is more appropriately described as "Osteitis". Infection of the periosteum alone should be called "periostitis".

○ **What are the common pathogens seen in osteomyelitis?**

Many studies have shown that Streptococcus species and Staphylococcus aureus were the most common pathogens in osteomyelitis. Anaerobes are not common, but when isolated were often gram-positive with Peptostreptococcus species most common. Bacteroides species are the most common gram-negative anaerobic organism in osteomyelitis.

○ **What is the etiology of pedal osteomyelitis?**

While neuropathic ulceration is the most common condition that can lead to pedal osteomyelitis, puncture wounds can easily lead to osteomyelitis if not treated properly. Hematogenous osteomyelitis is seen in children but is very rare in adults. Open fractures and post bony-surgery can be predisposed to osteomyelitis.

○ **Classification of osteomyelitis?**

There are two classification systems often used to classify osteomyelitis.

The Ciemy-Mader was developed to describe long bone osteomyelitis. It needs to be modified to describe pedal osteomyelitis. The system is based on the anatomy of the bone and the physiological status of the host. The Waldvogel classification is an etiologic system. Both systems can be used concurrently to effectively describe osteomyelitis and to develop treatment guidelines.

○ **Antibiotic therapy for osteomyelitis?**

Most authors agree that infection in patients with diabetes is poly-microbial. Patient should be started with an empiric broad-spectrum antibiotic. The medication may be adjusted based on results of wound and bone cultures. In most cases, intravenous antibiotics are more efficacious than oral antibiotics. The duration of antibiotic course is not clear. Most clinicians place patient on a six-week course, but the length can vary between 4 and 12 weeks.

○ **What need to be examined when evaluating diabetic patients with osteomyelitis?**

Examination of patients with possible osteomyelitis should not be deviated from any other type of physical examination. A careful history of the ulcer is extremely helpful. Even in the case of a severe infection, many of these patients will not relate any constitutional symptoms. Past medical and surgical history, allergy, current medications can help determine the appropriate course of treatment. Vital signs are important even though many diabetic patients will not mount fever in response to their infection. A finger stick to determine blood glucose may provide a clue to the severity of infection. A complete physical exam can provide information needed to chart a successful treatment plan. The ulcer and surrounding soft tissue need to be evaluated thoroughly. Any exposed bone is highly suggestive of osteomyelitis. The presence of sinus tract that can lead a metal probe to the underlying bone is also highly suggestive of osteomyelitis. Kidney function needs to be evaluated to dose the antimicrobial therapy properly. Blood cultures are not always necessary but needed if the patient appears septic. Radiographic examination may not provide much information about osteomyelitis but can provide good detail for any structural deformity.

○   **Role of Bone scan in diagnosis of osteomyelitis?**

The use of bone scans in diagnosing osteomyelitis has made strides in the past few years. The three-phase bone scan is highly sensitive but has a poor specificity. Many modifications have been made to improve the specificity. Techniques currently available or under investigation include: Technetium-99m (99m-Tc) methylene diphosphonate scanning, Gallium-67 scanning, Indium-111- (111-In) labeled leukocyte scanning, Technetium-99m hexamethylpropylene amine oxime (HMPAO)-labeled leukocyte scintigraphy, 99m-Tc/111n-human immunoglobin, antigranulocyte antibodies. These newer techniques have been shown to improve the sensitivity and specificity of the scan to over 90%. The difficulty encountered is that some procedures require drawing blood and re-introducing it into the patient. Some patients may not tolerate the radioactive-labeled material.

○   **Role of MRI in diagnosis of osteomyelitis?**

The advantage of MRI is that it is non-invasive but some patients may have claustrophobia and not able to undergo the procedure. MRI is becoming cheaper as technology advances and the sensitivity and specificity of the procedure has been reported to be close to 100% in some institutions.

○   **Other diagnosis modalities for osteomyelitis?**

Probing to bone appears to be the most cost-effective method to make the diagnosis of osteomyelitis. This method has been shown to have a good sensitivity and specificity. A recent unpublished study from the same institution shows sensitivity and specificity comparable to those of Magnetic Resonance Imaging and Bone scan. Ultrasound method is being evaluated for making diagnosis of osteomyelitis.

○   **Invasive diagnosis of osteomyelitis?**

The gold standard for making the diagnosis of osteomyelitis is bone pathology. Bone specimen can be obtained by biopsy. Bone culture from the biopsy can easily be contaminated yielding false results, but this should not affect the anti-microbial therapy because the organism that infected the soft tissue and the bone should be similar. If surgery is performed to remove the osteomyelitic bone, the specimen should always be sent to pathology for examination.

○   **Treatment for osteomyelitis?**

Because osteomyelitis is in most cases the extension of soft tissue infection, medical management should not be different from those provided to ulcer. Optimal management requires multidisciplinary approach. Medical conditions such as hyperglycemia, nephropathy, or cardiac insufficiency need to be addressed while treating the osteomyelitis. Antimicrobial therapy will help control and treat sepsis. The wound and any exposed bones needs to be debrided aggressively. The ulcerated area needs to be offloaded using the method(s) the provider is most experienced with. The wound bed should be kept cleansed and moist using appropriate wound care products. Any deficient circulation to the ulcer area needs to be restored for the ulcer and the bone to have a chance to heal. Surgical removal of the bone followed by delay secondary closure has been shown by many authors to be the most effective method to treat osteomyelitis. In some cases, skin graft, advancement flap, rotational flap, or free tissue transfer may be required to cover a large defect caused by the infected ulcer with osteomyelitis.

○   **What is sequestration?**

It is a segment of dead, devascularized bone due to Haversian and Volkman canal and osteocyte destruction. The process is highly suggestive of osteomyelitis. Diabetic neuropathic arthropathy may have similar presentation.

○   **What is involucrum?**

As the infection progresses, the periosteum is elevated by purulent material. The new bone formation under the periosteum is called involucrum. This is also suggestive of osteomyelitis.

○   **What is Cloaca?**

Cloaca is the formation seen at the bone-periosteal interface to extrude sequestmm and other necrotic products from the infected bone.

○   **How does peripheral vascular disease affect osteomyelitis?**

The presence of PVD must be recognized and treated for patients with osteomyelitis. If not treated, the disease will prolong hospitalization and may even lead to unnecessary amputation.

DIABETES AND INFECTIOUS DISEASES

○ **What are the pathogenic factors in diabetic foot ulcers?**

Infection, neuropathy, and ischemia.

○ **What are the typical signs of infection in diabetics?**

Inflammation, purulence, sinus tracts, crepitation, cellulitis, hyperglycemia are usually seen in association with foot infections. Do not rely on fever, chills, or leukocytosis since their absence has been reported in over two thirds of patients with limb threatening infections.

○ **What is a common sign of limb- or life-threatening infection?**

Hyperglycemia.

○ **What organisms are involved in mild diabetic foot infections?**

Aerobic gram-positive cocci such as Staphylococcus aureus or streptococcus.

○ **What organisms are involved in severe limb threatening infections?**

Polymicrobial infections usually involve aerobic gram-positive cocci (staph. or strep.), gram-negative bacilli (E. Coli, klebsiella species, or proteus species), and anaerobes (bacteroides species and Peptostreptococcus).

○ **In the diabetic foot, what diagnosis must be considered if redness, swelling, and warmth exist?**

Charcot disease must be ruled out unless obvious signs of infection.

○ **What is the preferred weightbearing status of an infected or noninfected neuropathic ulcer?**

Ideally avoidance of any weightbearing is preferred, however, realistically minimized pressure can be achieved with total contact casting or felted foam dressings in order to provide decreased pressure to the affected area and allow healing to occur.

○ **In the diabetic foot, what are the common signs of infection typically seen?**

Due to the diabetes, signs of local infection are often subtle and may not manifest until severe infection. Hyperglycemia and flu-like symptoms may be the only warning signs.

○ **What is the ultimate goal in the management of the diabetic foot?**

Prevention of ulceration or recurrent ulceration, which increases the patient's susceptibility to infection.

○ **What are the steps to preventing infection in the diabetic foot?**

Regular foot inspection with an emphasis on proper foot hygiene.

Daily shoe inspection including the changing of shoes after several hours to prevent repetitive pressure to a focal area.
Adequate control of the blood sugars, cessation of smoking, exercise, and periodic physician examination will assist in the avoidance of infection.

○ **What are the typical organisms seen in severe diabetic foot ulcers?**

In severe cases, polymicrobial infection with aerobic gram positive cocci, aerobic gram negative bacilli, and anaerobic isolates of gram negative and or gram positive bacteria.

○ **Name common organisms seen in diabetic foot infections.**

Staphylococcus aureus.
Staphylococcus epidermidis.
Streptococcus.
Enterococcus.
Escherichia coil.
Proteus species.
Bacteroides species.
Peptococcus.
Peptostreptococcus.
Clostridium.

○ **How does one select an antibiotic for a diabetic foot infection?**

One must first determine whether the infection is non limb threatening, limb threatening, or life threatening. This will allow for empirical coverage via expected pathogens. Then the patient's history, in terms of drug allergies, renal and liver functions must be determined prior to the onset of any antibiotic. When possible, wound cultures should be sent to microbiology to assist in the appropriate selection of antibiotics.

○ **When treating a diabetic foot infection with oral antibiotics, what must one consider?**

Diabetic gastropathy which may alter the absorption of any oral medication. Thus the antibiotic serum levels may be less than adequate for eradication.

○ **What is the initial treatment of a limb or life-threatening diabetic foot infection?**

Early incision and drainage with debridement of all necrotic soft tissue and bone.

○ **What is the initial treatment of a non-limb-threatening diabetic foot infection?**

Pending a thorough examination of the diabetic foot, one's clinical judgment will determine whether the wound is non-limb-threatening versus limb/life-threatening. Provided the wound is deemed non-limb-threatening, an antibiotic course of therapy can begin.

○ **What is the most important risk factor for ulceration in the diabetic foot? and how can one slow the progression?**

Neuropathy is the major factor in which glycemic control can slow its progression.

○ **What is the management of osteomyelitis in the diabetic foot?**

Upon diagnosis through radiographs, sterile bone probes, bone scans, CT scans, or MRI's, the infected bone must be debrided or limited amputation. A two-three week course of antibiotics will follow to eliminate any remaining soft tissue infection.

CHARCOT FOOT DEFORMITY

○ **Provide five synonyms for Charcot foot.**

Neuropathic osteoarthropathy, diabetic neuroarthropathy, Charcot's arthropathy, neuropathic arthropathy.

○ **Define Charcot joint disease.**

Charcot constitutes a highly destructive and relatively painless disorder that involves singular or multiple joints.

○ **What is the original disorder associated with Charcot joint disease?**

Jean Martin Charcot in 1868 described neuropathic joint changes in patients with tabes dorsalis.

○ **What is the current disorder associated with Charcot joint disease?**

In 1936 Jordan was the first to associate neuropathic arthropathy with diabetes mellitus, which has emerged as the primary cause with the declining incidence of tertiary syphilis.

○ **Name the four most common disorders with potential for neuropathic osteoarthropathy.**

Diabetes mellitus, tertiary syphilis, leprosy, and syringomyelia.

○ **Besides the four most common disorders related with Charcot joint disease, name ten other potential causes.**

Spina bifida, meningomyelocele, congenital insensitivity to pain, hysterical insensitivity to pain, chronic alcoholism, peripheral nerve injury, sciatic nerve severance, spinal cord injury, myelodysplasia, poliomyelitis, multiple sclerosis, Riley-Day syndrome, intra-articular injections, and paraplegia.

○ **Name four diseases causing neuropathic osteoarthropathy with predilection for the foot and ankle.**

Diabetes mellitus, leprosy, meningomyelocele, and congenital insensitivity to pain.

○ **What is the pathogenesis for Charcot joint disease?**

Although unclear it is multifactorial. Two theories attributed to the pathogenesis are the neurotraumatic and neurovascular reflex theory. The former relies on neuropathy and repeated trauma, which produces the eventual joint destruction. The latter proposes increased peripheral blood flow from autonomic neuropathy, which results in abundant bone resorption.

○ **Who provided the radiographic staging used in neuropathic osteoarthropathy? Describe the stages.**

The radiographic stages of development, coalescence, and reconstruction were described by Eichenholtz in 1966. The development stage has initial destruction consisting of joint laxity, subluxation, osteochondral fragmentation and debris formation. The coalescence has absorption of debris and fusion of fragments to adjacent bone. The stage of reconstruction increases stabilization by trabecular remodeling, osseous proliferation and ankylosis.

○ **What are the clinical features of an acute Charcot deformity?**

The classic findings involve the vascular, neuropathic, skeletal, and cutaneous status of the patient. The pulses are usually bounding with warmth, swelling, and erythema. There is always some degree of neuropathy with reduced or absent reflexes, proprioception, vibratory sense, and/or pain. Autonomic neuropathy in the form of anhydrosis is seen. The skeletal system provides hypermobility and crepitus resulting in some pedal deformity resulting in some pedal deformity such as rocker bottom. The severity of the skeletal deformity allows cutaneous lesions such as hyperkeratoses or ulcerations, which create the potential for infection.

○ **Name five differential diagnoses for Charcot joint disease.**

Acute septic arthritis, gout, rheumatoid arthritis, psoriatic arthritis, osteoarthritis, tuberculous arthritis, paraplegia, and neoplasms.

○ **What is the mainstay for treatment of acute neuropathic arthropathy?**

Conservative therapy by cessation of weightbearing of the involved extremity in order to prevent further destruction.

○ **What is the Sanders classification of neuropathic osteoarthropathy?**

Sanders and Mrdjencovich describe the Charcot patterns based upon the location in diabetic patients.

Pattern I:	Forefoot
Pattern II:	Tarsometatarsals
Pattern III:	Midtarsal and Naviculocuneiform
Pattern IV:	Ankle and Subtalar joint
Pattern V:	Calcaneus (Posterior pillar)

○ **Which pattern of the Sanders classification may in fact not be neuropathic osteoarthropathy?**

Pattern V involves fractures of the calcaneus but does not involve any joints. This has been referred to as a calcaneal insufficiency fracture or simply a neuropathic fracture.

○ **Name three immobilizers used in the care of acute Charcot with deep ulceration.**

Typically these are removable modalities to allow dressing changes and close inspection of the wound. A bivalve cast, CAM walker, or Charcot restraint orthotic walker (CROW).

○ **What is the conservative treatment of a patient in the coalescent stage of rearfoot Charcot?**

Depending upon the severity of the deformity different modalities exist. For mild ankle deformity a high top custom molded shoe may suffice. The moderately unstable ankle deformity a solid ankle foot orthoses (AFO) and a therapeutic shoe should provide enough support. The severely unstable ankle will need a patellar tendon bearing brace in a custom shoe.

○ **What are the indications for surgical reconstruction of the Charcot foot?**

Marked instability and recalcitrant ulceration.

○ **What adjunctive procedure is usually performed with rearfoot Charcot reconstructions?**

Commonly the tendo Achilles is lengthened in order to reduce the equinus deformity, which often exists. Otherwise if the ankle is to be fused then the release of the Achilles tendon allows greater ease achieving optimal positioning.

○ **What are the goals of Charcot reconstruction?**

The goal is a plantigrade foot with the ankle at 90 degrees, the hindfoot in 5-10 degrees of valgus rotation, and external rotation equivalent to the opposite foot.

EMERGENCY MEDICINE

○ **A patient complains of chest pain that is aching in nature and tender to pressure and movement. What is the most likely etiology of the chest pain?**

Musculoskeletal.

○ **Describe the changes seen on the ECG that suggest a high probability for acute myocardial infarction.**

ST segment elevation greater than 1mm in 2 contiguous leads and new Q waves.

○ **What is Anaphylaxis?**

A severe allergic reaction involving multiple organ systems, which occurs in an individual who has had prior sensitization to an antigen and with later reexposure, produces symptoms via an immunologic mechanism.

○ **Discuss the difference between an anaphylactic reaction and an anaphylactoid reaction.**

Anaphylaxis produces symptoms via an immunologic mechanism whereas an anaphylactoid reaction produces a very similar clinical picture but is not immune-mediated. Treatment of both conditions is similar.

○ **Describe the clinical manifestations seen in an anaphylactic reaction.**

Cutaneous manifestations include urticaria, erythema, pruritus, and angioedema. Respiratory manifestations include nasal congestion, sneezing, coughing, hoarseness, tightness of the throat, dyspnea. Cardiovascular manifestations include hypotension with resultant weakness, dizziness or syncope, chest pain, myocardial ischemia. Gastrointestinal manifestations include abdominal pain with nausea, vomiting or diarrhea.

○ **What is syncope?**

A sudden transient loss of consciousness usually due to transient cerebral hypoperfusion.

○ **What are the types of shock?**

Hypovolemic, Cardiogenic, Distributive (includes septic shock, neurogenic shock, anaphylactic shock), obstructive shock.

○ **Describe the local manifestations seen with toxicity of local anesthetics.**

Neurovascular manifestations such as prolonged anesthesia and paresthesia (may become irreversible).

○ **Describe the pathophysiologic mechanism of anaphylaxis.**

After exposure to an inciting substance, this antigen (allergen) binds to antigen-specific IgE that had been attached to previously sensitized basophils and mast cells. Mediators are released almost immediately when the antigen binds which cause the effects seen in anaphylaxis.

○ **Describe the pathophysiologic mechanism of an anaphylactoid reaction.**

Exposure to an inciting substance causes direct release of mediators, a process not mediated by IgE.

O   **Describe the signs and symptoms that may occur with hypoglycemia.**

Headache, confusion, personality changes, nausea, hunger, sweating, anxiety, tremors, nervousness, faintness, weakness, palpitations, tachycardia.

O   **What are the signs and symptoms of acute myocardial infarction?**

Severe, prolonged chest pain, described as tightness, pressure, or squeezing (may radiate to jaw, neck, arms (Left >Right), back, and epigastrium), SOB, weakness, nausea, vomiting anxiety, lightheadedness, syncope, cough, diaphoresis.

O   **Describe the upper respiratory versus lower respiratory effects that can occur in an anaphylactic reaction.**

Severe upper airway obstruction by angioedema can lead to asphyxia while lower airway obstruction with wheezing and chest tightness is caused by bronchospasm.

O   **What is vasovagal syncope?**

Precipitated by stress or pain, a reflex vagal bradycardia and peripheral vasodilatation causing decreased cerebral blood flow.

O   **What does Flumazenil do?**

Reverses effect of Benzodiazepines.

O   **How soon can clinical manifestations of anaphylaxis occur after exposure to an antigen?**

Clinical manifestations can occur within seconds of antigen exposure.

O   **Is Flumazenil used as an empiric treatment in the comatose patient? Why?**

No. It may induce seizures in patients who have also taken tricyclic antidepressants or other convulsants and may interfere with the later use of benzodiazepines to manage seizures.

O   **List the signs and symptoms seen with local anesthetic toxicity.**

Initially see lightheadedness, dizziness, visual and auditory disturbances, disorientation, drowsiness. At higher doses often see initial CNS excitation followed by a rapid CNS depression, muscle twitching, convulsions, unconsciousness, coma, respiratory depression and arrest, cardiovascular depression and collapse. Other signs and symptoms include chest pain, SOB, palpitations, diaphoresis, hypotension, syncope, methemoglobinemia.

O   **What are the mediators involved in an anaphylactic reaction?**

 Histamine, leukotriene C4, prostaglandin D2, and tryptase.

O   **Of the two groups of local anesthetics, which is more likely to cause an allergic reaction and why?**

Amino-esters. They are derivatives of para-aminobenzoic acid (PABA), which has been associated with acute allergic reactions. NB: Amino-amides are not associated with PABA and do not produce manifest allergic reactions with the same frequency. However, sometimes these contain Methylparaben, which is structurally similar to PABA and can result in an allergic reaction.

❍ **A patient has an allergic reaction to a local anesthetic in your office. What is the pharmacological treatment?**

Mild cutaneous reactions may be treated with Benadryl (25-50 mg IV/ PO for adult doses and 1.0 mg/kg for pediatric doses). Patients with more serious reactions should be treated with 0.3 cc of SQ epinephrine (1:1000) and receive close monitoring.

❍ **Describe mild, moderate and severe hypertension.**

Mild – diastolic 90-104, Moderate – diastolic 105-114, Severe – diastolic > 115

❍ **Name the agent that is widely used as an empiric antidote for any patient with suspected opiate intoxication.**

Naloxone.

❍ **What are some noncardiac causes of Sudden Death?**

CNS hemorrhage, massive PE, drug overdose, hypoxia secondary to lung disease, aortic dissection or rupture.

❍ **What is the most common cause of septic shock?**

Gram-negative bacterial infection – related to the release of endotoxin (part of bacterial cell wall).

❍ **What is the most common cause of sudden cardiac death?**

Ventricular tachyarrhythmias, generally related to ischemic heart disease.

❍ **Describe the clinical manifestations seen with a vasovagal reaction.**

Pallor, malaise, dizziness and light- headedness, nausea, diaphoresis, increased salivation, and syncope.

❍ **List the five "P"s seen in acute arterial occlusion.**

Pain, paralysis, paresthesia, pallor, pulselessness.

❍ **What are the most commonly reported medical agents causing anaphylaxis?**

Penicillin and cephalosporin antibiotics.

❍ **Discuss the stages of shock.**

Stage I: "Compensated hypotension" – fall in cardiac output or in the delivery of cardiac output to tissues stimulates a variety of compensatory mechanisms that alter myocardial function and peripheral resistance to maintain circulation to vital organs. The clinical symptoms in the stage are minimal.

Stage II: Compensatory mechanisms for dealing with low delivery of nutrients to body are overwhelmed and tissue perfusion is decreased. Early signs of cerebral, renal and myocardial insufficiency can occur. If treatment occurs, recovery is still probable in this stage.

Stage III: Tissues and organs begin to suffer permanent damage from lack of Oxygen. Organs fail as progress through this stage. End result is death.

❍   **How does position affect a patient with a vasovagal reaction?**

Symptoms improve promptly with recumbency (will disappear altogether without treatment in 20-30 minutes).

❍   **What are the three end organs most commonly affected in a hypertensive emergency?**

Brain, heart and kidneys.

❍   **What are the two categories of seizure?**

Partial seizure – discrete area of brain (may secondarily involve rest of brain) and Generalized seizure involving simultaneous onset from both hemispheres.

❍   **What blood work should be ordered for a comatose patient?**

This should include CBC, BUN, creatinine, glucose, electrolytes, calcium, toxicology, and ABGs.

❍   **What is N-acetylcysteine?**

Antidote to acetaminophen toxicity – most effective if administered within 8-10 hrs.

❍   **What else is given along with IV glucose in the comatose patient? Why?**

Thiamine should be given with IV glucose. Glucose alone will increase thiamine utilization, and worsen patients with thiamine deficiency (Wernicke's encephalopathy).

❍   **What is the most common cause of local anesthetic toxicity?**

Inadvertent intravascular injection.

❍   **Describe malignant hyperthermia?**

Disorder of muscle cells leading to sustained rigidity after certain stimuli (usually succinylcholine, halothane, or other general anesthetics). It is inherited as an autosomal recessive genetic abnormality.

❍   **What is malignant or accelerated hypertension?**

Rapidly progressive and aggressive disease characterized by severe elevation in BP associated with widespread end organ dysfunction.

❍   **What is the most common type of shock?**

Hypovolemic.

❍   **What is the first priority with a comatose patient?**

Be sure the patient is breathing, and if breathing is not adequate, establish an airway and maintain respiration. After this, measure BP, establish IV access and draw blood for testing.

❍   **What is the gold standard for detection on myocardial infarction?**

CPK-MB (creatinine phosphokinase).

❍ **Name the mainstay of pharmacologic treatment administered as first-line therapy for severe anaphylaxis when systemic manifestations occur.**

Epinephrine.

❍ **How is the above drug typically administered and what is the dosage?**

It is given subcutaneously, 0.3-0.5 ml 1:1000 soln. Q15 min except for patients with life threatening reactions with shock involved for whom it is given IV, 1.0 ml 1:10.000 soln (diluted in 10ccNS) slow IV, repeat prn. Sublingual form is available.

❍ **What are some other common pharmacologic agents used in the treatment of anaphylaxis?**

Diphenhydramine HCL, 50 mg PO, IM, or IV, Methylprednisolone sodium succinate, 125 mg IV, Bronchodilators (inhaled beta2 agonists, IV aminophylline), Vasopressors (norepinephrine or dopamine HCL), Histamine2 antagonists, Glucagon *, Atropine sulfate *, isoproterenol *
*Useful in refractory anaphylaxis induced by beta-blocker therapy.

❍ **What is the maximum dosage guide for lidocaine (Xylocaine)?**

4.5 mg/kg without epinephrine and 7 mg/kg with epinephrine.
(The minimum dose of lidocaine at which adverse reactions occurred is 6.4 mg/kg).

❍ **What is the maximum dosage guide for bupivacaine (Marcaine)?**

175 mg without Epi and 225 mg with Epi.
(The minimum dose of bupivacaine at which adverse reactions occurred is 1.6 mg/kg).

❍ **What is the most common cause of death in anaphylaxis?**

Complete airway obstruction from edema.

❍ **What is the most effective IV agent available for rapid blood pressure control?**

Na Nitroprusside.

❍ **While anesthetizing a toe, Epinephrine is inadvertently injected and the toe turns white. What is the treatment?**

Dependent position of foot, warm compresses to proximal NV bundle, vasodilatory patches proximal to area, local blocks proximal to area, vascular consult.

❍ **What is the treatment for a patient with malignant hyperthermia?**

Dantrolene - acts directly on the muscle cell, evaporative cooling may also help.

❍ **What physical exam finding is pathognomonic for hypertensive encephalopathy?**

Papilledema.

❍ **Why can glucose be administered to a comatose patient without knowing the cause of unconsciousness?**

Glucose may be life saving in patients with hypoglycemia and it will do little to worsen patients with hyperglycemic hyperosmolar coma.

○   Describe the compressions to breaths ratio in one versus two man CPR.

One man CPR – 15 compressions/ 2 breaths; two man CPR – 5 compressions/ 1 breath.

○   What is the most common cause of airway obstruction in the unconscious person?

The tongue.

○   What is the rate of chest compressions in an infant?

At least 100 times per minute (newborn 120/minute).

○   What maneuver is done to open an airway? If the patient is a trauma victim, how does this change?

Head tilt – chin lift if no trauma. If there is trauma, use jaw thrust.

○   Describe where one would check the pulse in the unconscious adult, child, and infant.

In child (1 to 8 years old) and adult, check the carotid pulse. In an infant, check the brachial or femoral pulse.

○   Describe the hand position when performing chest compressions on an adult.

One hand is placed on top of the other with the heel of the lower hand pressing over the lower half of the sternum.

○   What maneuvers are done for a choking infant?

Back Blows (5) and chest thrusts (5).

INTERNAL FIXATION

○ **Which type of bone are staples designed for, Cortical or Cancellous?**

Cancellous.

○ **Do you typically find callous formation with rigid internal fixation?**

No, this generally indicates motion at the fracture/osteotomy site.

○ **For fixation of an oblique fracture, should the screw fixation be perpendicular to the long axis of the bone or to the fracture line?**

To the bone (cortex); this will prevent movement sliding of the fragments on each other during axial loading.

○ **What is the special design of a Herbert bone screw?**

It has no head and the pitch of the threads on either end of the screw is different from each other.

○ **Should plate fixation lie on the compression side or on the tension side?**

Tension.

○ **When utilizing plate fixation on a fracture, the screw should be located where on the screw hole?**

Eccentrically, away from the fracture site.

○ **Name another fixation method, which provides compression across a fracture line.**

Tension band wire.

○ **What is the fixation device of choice for a fracture with soft tissue loss?**

External fixation.

○ **Why is the proximal cortex over drilled when using lag technique?**

To prevent distraction of the osteotomy and allow for compression.

○ **What is the difference between cortical and cancellous screws?**

The pitch of the screw (cortical is 1.25mm & cancellous is 1.75mm).

○ **Lag technique is necessary when using a cannulated, partially threaded, cancellous screw. T or F?**

False. Because this is a partially threaded screw, only the threads (which are distal to the fracture/osteotomy) will purchase the bone and compression will still be achieved.

○ **During placement of a 2.7mm cortical screw with lag technique, you accidentally over drill the far side of bone in relation to your osteotomy. What is your next best option?**

Go up to the next larger size screw.

○ **The Ilizarov bone lengthening osteotomy requires how long of a period of compression before callous distraction begins?**

Three weeks.

○ **What is the maximum documented amount of callous distraction that can be achieved in one day with the Ilizarov bone lengthening procedure?**

1mm.

○ **What is the first step in proper lag technique?**

Reduce the fracture / osteotomy with a bone clamp.

○ **What is the number one complication of an external fixator?**

Infection.

○ **What should you do if you break the suture off of a Mitek≤ bone Anchor?**

Stop shouting, trephine out the anchor, or leave it, and insert a new anchor in a different location.

○ **(T or F) K-wires offer compression when crossed?**

False, K-wires provide splintage but not compression.

○ **Is secondary bone healing (gap healing) a principle of standard internal fixation?**

No, rigid internal fixation allows for primary bone healing (contact healing).

○ **What is an absolute contraindication for the use of internal fixation?**

Infection.

○ **According to internal fixation technique, how many cortices must a single trans-syndesmotic screw cross when there is disruption of the distal tibial-fibular syndesmosis?**

4 cortices.

○ **What is the most appropriate form of fixation used for an end to end arthrodesis of a PIPJ?**

A K-wire retrograded from distal to proximal.

○ **What is the most appropriate method of fixation for a Salter Harris type IV fracture of the distal tibia?**

Smooth K-wire.

○ **The weakest segment of a screw is?**

The run out, which is where the shaft meets the core. The core of the screw is the portion of the shaft that extends into the thread pattern. The shaft of the screw is portion without a thread pattern.

○ **Why is it important to countersink when using screw fixation?**

Countersinking reduces the prominence of the screw head. It also increases the surface area between the cortex and the screw head, which serves to prevent stress risers. It also creates a concentric relationship with the thread hole, which prevents lateral movement of the head of the screw as it engages the cortex.

○ **Which type of fixation causes the best compression?**

Screw fixation.

○ **Which method of fixation would be most advantageous in opening wedge osteotomies?**

Staples because they maintain the size of the osteotomy when bone graft is being resorbed.

○ **The term "cutting cone" refers to?**

Osteons, which cross the fracture line. Each remodeling osteon is composed of leading osteoclasts which create a resorption canal that is then invaded by vascular buds. Circumferentially oriented osteoblasts then give rise to new osteon.

○ **What would you expect to be the cause, if you observed a radiograph with callus formation about the osteotomy site, with fixation in place?**

Motion at the site.

○ **List two reasons that a delayed union may occur?**

Inadequate alignment and apposition of the fracture fragments at the time of reduction. Motion at the osteotomy site.

○ **A malunion is defined as?**

Inadequate positional healing of an osteotomy or fracture site.

○ **How long should a patient remain non-weight bearing following a base osteotomy of the first metatarsal?**

Six to eight weeks.

○ **What is the most inherently stable fracture pattern?**

Transverse type.

○ **What is the complication of not over drilling the proximal fragment in standard AO screw fixation?**

It causes distraction rather than compression.

○ **The correct sequence for the insertion of a 3.5mm cortical screw?**

2.5mm threaded hole, countersink, 3.5mm gliding hole, depth gauge, tap3.5mm, apply screw

❍   **When fixating a fracture, is the "load screw" perpendicular to the bone or is it perpendicular to the fracture.**

Perpendicular to the bone.

❍   **When using single screw technique to fixate a closing base wedge osteotomy describe the orientation of the screw.**

Equal distance between the perpendicular to the long axis of the bone and the perpendicular to the fracture line.

❍   **A 27 y/o man develops a foot infection three weeks after open reduction and internal fixation of a pilon ankle fracture with interfragmentary screws and a medial buttress plate. The wound is débrided to bone; in this case should the hardware be left in place or removed?**

Removed.

❍   **What is the pitch of a cancellous screw?**

1.75.

❍   **How many threads of the screw should extend beyond the far cortex?**

Two.

❍   **Theoretically, a fixation plate used on a transverse midshaft fracture of a metatarsal should be placed where?**

On the plantar aspect of the metatarsal which is the side of tension.

❍   **A contraindication to *Grafton®* (Allogenic bone grafting gel) would be?**

A history of a Bacitracin allergy.

❍   **How long will an *OrthoSorb®* (polydioxanone) pin retain it's strength?**

4-8 weeks, absorbed in 9-12 weeks.

❍   **Name the three forces affecting stability of fracture reduction?**

Bending, shear, torsion.

❍   **In terms of screws, the "land" refers to what part of a screw?**

Undersurface of the screw head.

❍   **What type of screw, cancellous or cortical, is generally accepted for use in the calcaneous?**

Cancellous.

❍   **When can a screw be used alone for internal fixation of a fracture?**

When the fracture is at least twice as long as the diameter of the bone at the level of the fracture.

○ **The tension band principle is an example of what type of compression?**

Dynamic compression.

○ **The best type of fixation for pseudoarthrosis, following bone debridement and graft placement is?**

Neutralization plates.

○ **Pneumatic surgical instruments use which type of gas?**

Nitrogen.

○ **Which clinical symptom indicates a possible malunion?**

Prolonged swelling, angulation at the fracture/osteotomy site, pain and stiffness.

○ **Which type of screw fixation allows for percutaneous placement across a fracture site?**

Cannulated.

○ **The most common complication when using external K-wires is ?**

Infection (pin tract).

○ **What is the minimum number of K-wires needed to achieve frontal plane stability of a distal metaphyseal osteotomy?**

Two, unless the osteotomy has inherent frontal plane stability (an Austin osteotomy for instance) in which case one K-wire may suffice.

○ **What is the purpose of a Jones cast?**

Reduction of edema through compression.

○ **One of the primary reasons to use external fixation is:**

Immediate weight bearing.

○ **Prebending of a plate provides for?**

Uniform compression at the osteotomy site.

○ **Contraindications to open reduction internal fixation (ORIF) include?**

Peripheral vascular disease, infection, open contaminated injuries, extensive soft tissue damage, significant bone loss.

○ **(T or F) A neutralization plate produces interfragmentary compression?**

False.

○ **Which fracture pattern is least stable?**

Comminuted.

O   **According to Pauwels principal, a long bone eccentrically loaded is subjected to tension forces on the convex side and what force on the concave side?**

Compression forces.

O   **Which effect is produced, when using two different types of metals in close proximity to each other within the body.**

Galvanic corrosion (a battery effect).

O   **The basic techniques of internal fixation are?**

Splinting, neutralization, buttressing, interfragmentary compression.

O   **Which thread diameter is larger in general, a cortical or cancellous screw?**

Cancellous.

O   **(T or F) The use of plates and screws allows for the postoperative patient to ambulate in a weight-bearing attitude?**

False, AO fixation is meant allow joint movement (prevents cast disease) but is not meant to withstand weight-bearing forces.

O   **What is a transfixation screw used for?**

Used to approximate the fibula to the tibia when an interosseous ligament rupture (diastasis) occurs.

O   **If a patient relates a nickel allergy, what would be the best choice to fixate a closing base wedge osteotomy?**

Bio-Absorbable screw.

O   **What is the primary advantage of a screw has over a K-wire, when fixating an osteotomy site?**

The screw provides compression.

O   **What is not expected to be seen radiographically, at an osteotomy site, with screw fixation, 5 weeks postop?**

Callous formation.

O   **When observing a radiograph at 5 weeks out, sclerosis is noted at the osteotomy site what would be a likely possible explanation?**

The beginning of a non-union.

O   **What would be appropriate to use when reattaching the Achilles tendon back onto the calcaneus?**

A bone anchor system.

❍ **When reducing an oblique, midshaft fracture on the second metatarsal, which would be a better screw to use, a cortical or a cancellous?**

Cortical.

❍ **Do lag screws provide dynamic interfragmental compression?**

No, they provide static interfragmental compression.

❍ **How is dynamic interfragmental compression achieved? Give an example of its use in the foot.**

Dynamic interfragmental compression is achieved by the use of tension band fixation. Tension bands harness forces generated at the level of the fracture when the skeleton comes under physiological load. 5th metatarsal, styloid fractures can be fixated in this way.

❍ **What is the core diameter of a 4.0 mm cancellous screw?**

1.9 mm.

❍ **What is the size of the pilot hole needed to apply a 4.0 mm cancellous screw?**

2.5 mm.

❍ **What is the size of the tap needed to apply a 4.0 mm cancellous screw.**

3.5 mm.

❍ **What is the size of the pilot hole needed to apply a 2.7 mm cortical screw?**

2.0 mm.

❍ **What is the size of the tap needed to apply a 2.7 mm cortical screw?**

2.7 mm tap.

❍ **What is the size of the drill bit used to "over-drill" the proximal cortex when applying a 2.7 mm cortex?**

2.7 mm drill.

❍ **When are metal or ceramic washers possibly indicated?**

When utilizing screw fixation on soft, osteopenic bone or when reattaching avulsed soft tissue structures such as ligament or tendon to bone.

❍ **What is the primary function of a neutralization plate?**

To protect interfragmental compression lag screws from bending, shearing, and torsional forces.

❍ **What is the primary purpose of a buttress plate?**

To prevent axial deformity from bending, shearing and torsional forces.

❍ **What is the purpose of a posterior 1/3 semi-tubular plate in a distal oblique fibular fracture?**

This anti-glide plate prevents proximal migration of the distal fracture fragment.

O   **What is fracture disease?**

A clinical state, which is manifested by chronic edema, soft tissue atrophy, osteoporosis, and joint stiffness.

O   **What is the principle of the lag screw?**

The thread must not cross the fracture line.

O   **What is the principle of the tension band?**

The implant absorbs the tension and the bone the compression.

O   **What is the screw fixation principle?**

Two small screws obtain a better fixation than one large screw.

O   **What is the "Vassal Rule"?**

Where there is mechanical dependence between two fractures, the dominant fracture should be reduced first, after which the vassal fracture will reduce spontaneously or can be reduced easily. Only the dominant fracture requires a plate.

O   **What is the average time interval between internal fixation and removal of a screw from a metatarsal or hallux assuming normal healing has occurred?**

Screws should generally be removed within 4-6 months.

O   **What are the prerequisites for primary bone healing?**

Excellent anatomic alignment with rigid internal compression, complete immobilization, along with adequate vascularity.

O   **What are the common sizes of K-wires?**

0.035 inches, 0.045 inches, 0.054 inches, 0.062 inches.

O   **What is the most common size of stainless steel monofilament wire used in podiatric surgery?**

26 or 28 gauge.

O   **What are the common sizes of Steinmann pins used in podiatric surgery?**

5/64 – 3/16 inches.

O   **Which is stronger, a 0.045 inch smooth K-wire or a 0.045 in threaded K-wire?**

The smooth K-wire is stronger. The threaded K-wire has a thinner core and is therefore weaker.

O   **When applying bone screws, should the depth gauge be used prior to tapping or subsequent to tapping? Why?**

Always prior to tapping. Once the threads are tapped, the use of a depth gauge could disrupt the threads.

❍   **What is the shape of the recess in 1.5 mm and 2.0 mm Synthes mini cortex screw heads?**

Cruciate.

❍   **What is the shape of the recess in the 2.7 mm Synthes cortical and 4.0 mm Synthes cancellous screw heads?**

Hexagonal.

FLATFOOT

○ **A patient presents with a flexible pes valgus deformity. What would you expect to see on Clinical examination?**

Everted heel, abduction of forefoot on the rearfoot, collapse of the medial column, flexibility of the foot with reducibility of the deformity, foot functioning maximally pronated through gait cycle with little or no resupination, posterior equinus (most probable).

○ **What compensation occurs with equinus in a pes valgus foot?**

Early heel off, subtalar joint and midtarsal joint pronation, medial column sag, tarsometatarsal breech.

○ **Describe the biomechanical mechanism involved with compensation for equinus in a pes valgus foot.**

Ankle equinus prevents dorsiflexion of the talus, which maintains its position while the remainder of the foot (including calcaneus and navicular) dorsiflex, abduct, and evert from beneath it. This leads to a subluxatory collapse of the rearfoot on the forefoot.

○ **If transverse plane deformity dominates, which calcaneal osteotomy would be indicated?**

Evans calcaneal osteotomy.

○ **X-rays of a patient with pes valgus reveal a widening of the lesser tarsal area on the DP view, decrease of the first metatarsal declination angle, decrease of the height of sustentaculum tali, and increased superimposition of the lesser tarsal area on the lateral view. What is the dominant plane of deformity?**

Frontal plane.

○ **A patient with a unilateral flatfoot deformity unable to perform the single-limb heel-rise test. Diagnosis?**

Posterior tibial dysfunction or rupture.

○ **Axis-altering arthroereisis devices (ie. STA-peg) are used for flatfoot exhibiting primarily what plane of deformity?**

Frontal plane.

○ **Calcaneal osteotomies are classified (by Jacobs and associates) into three groups. Name the groups.**

extra-articular, anterior, and posterior osteotomies.

○ **Name the procedures in each category above.**

Extra-articular = Chambers, Baker-Hill, Selakovich.
Anterior = Evans.
Posterior = Gleich, Dwyer, Silver, Koutsogiannis.

○ **What are some causes of rigid pronated feet?**

Congenital convex pes plano valgus (vertical talus), improperly corrected clubfoot, tarsal coalition, peroneal spastic flatfoot, trauma, late stages of neuropathy.

○   **Describe the average axis of the STJ as originally described.**

42 degrees up from the transverse plane and 16 degrees from the sagittal plane. This allows approximately equal amounts of Frontal Plane motion as well as Transverse Plane motion.

○   **What is the Hubscher maneuver?**

While the patient is in relaxed stance, the hallux is passively dorsiflexed to determine the flexibility of the arch. With passive dorsiflexion, the windlass effect is invoked, and this tightens the medial band of the plantar fascia and long flexor of the hallux increasing the height of the arch.

○   **What is the Kidner procedure.**

Resection of the accessory navicular and any hypertrophy of the tuberosity, transposition of the insertion of the tibialis posterior tendon into the underside of the navicular.

○   **Describe the Young procedure.**

Rerouting tibialis anterior tendon through a slot in the navicular without detaching the tendon from its insertion, tibialis posterior reattachment beneath the navicular bone, TAL if needed.

○   **Describe the midtarsal joint when the subtalar joint is in its maximally pronated position with the calcaneus everted?**

Talonavicular and calcaneocuboid joints become divergent from each other with their axes more parallel allowing full, independent range of motion of each of these joints and increasing the range of motion of the MTJ itself.

○   **Where is the osteotomy made for the Evans procedure?**

Approximately 1.5 cm proximal and parallel to the C-C joint.

○   **How is this osteotomy (Evans) directed and why?**

Directed anteriorly to avoid the middle facet of the STJ.

○   **Name possible etiologies of flexible pes valgus (underlying causes of excessive pronation)?**

Compensated forefoot varus, compensated flexible forefoot valgus, rearfoot equinus, congenital talipes calcaneovalgus, torsional abnormalities of adduction or abduction, muscle imbalance, ligamentous laxity, neurotrophic feet, medial shift in WB (i.e. obesity).

○   **During gait, the talus and the leg internally rotate and adduct to take up motion in what plane?**

Transverse plane.

○   **What incisional approach is necessary when performing a triple arthrodesis for pes valgus?**

Two-incision approach used to afford adequate access to the midtarsal and subtalar joints.

○   **Describe the Dwyer osteotomy.**

Opening wedge with bone graft in lateral calcaneus (more common) or closing wedge in medial calcaneus (closing wedge can be performed in a large heel).

○ **How is congenital calcaneovalgus deformity easily distinguished from congenital convex pes plano valgus deformity on clinical examination?**

Congenital calcaneovalgus is flexible and allows for passive correction.

○ **How much dorsiflexion at the ankle joint is necessary during a normal gait cycle to avoid compensation for limitation of motion?**

10 degrees.

○ **If the STJ axis fell parallel to the transverse plane, motion around the axis would primarily be in what plane?**

Frontal plane.

○ **If the STJ axis is more vertical for an individual, what plane of motion will be dominant?**

Transverse plane motion.

○ **Imbalance or dysfunction of what muscle will quickly lead to a pes valgus deformity?**

Tibialis posterior.

○ **In a flexible pes valgus deformity, describe what happens to the foot (ie 1st ray, rearfoot, etc.) when the Hubscher maneuver is performed. How would this compare to a patient with a tarsal coalition?**

Plantarflexion of 1st ray, supination of RF, external rotation of leg, significant increase in height of medial arch. In tarsal coalition, foot would fail to show response.

○ **When weight bearing, eversion of the calcaneus and foot take up motion in what plane?**

Frontal plane.

○ **What deformity cannot be present if the Evans procedure is planned?**

Metatarsus Adductus.

○ **What is the consequence if the Evans is performed in a foot with the above deformity?**

Unmasking and exaggeration of the metatarsus adductus and an in-toe gait.

○ **In patients under 1 year of age, what is one of the most common forerunners of pes valgus deformity?**

Congenital calcaneovalgus deformity.

○ **Describe the incision when performing the Kidner procedure.**

Dorsally arched longitudinal incision extending along the dorsomedial side of the foot from below the tip of the medial malleolus to the midshaft of the first metatarsal.

○   **Name the muscles and tendons visible in dissection when performing the Young's procedure.**

Tibialis anterior tendon, tibialis posterior tendon, abductor hallucis muscle.

○   **What muscle will be encountered when performing the Evans procedure?**

EDB muscle belly.

○   **Where is the bone graft inserted when doing the Evans procedure?**

Distal 1/3 of the calcaneus.

○   **How is the calcaneal inclination angle affected with positional changes of pronation and supination in the normal foot? How does this compare to the pes valgus foot?**

Normal foot changes very little. Calcaneo-Inclination Angle in pes valgus foot will be structurally lowered by subluxation of the rearfoot on the forefoot over a period of time.

○   **Instability of which column of the foot is more indicative of a pathological flatfoot condition?**

Lateral column.

○   **Ligamentous laxity can occur due to a defect in collagen synthesis. Name these disorders.**

Ehlers-Danlos syndrome, Marfan's syndrome, and osteogenesis imperfecta.

○   **What are the radiographic manifestations for a pes valgus deformity with sagittal plane dominance?**

Increased talar declination angle, naviculocuneiform breach, increased talocalcaneal angle on lateral view, decreased Calcaneo-Inclination Angle.

○   **Name some abduction deformities of the lower extremity that can lead to a flexible pes valgus deformity?**

Metatarsus abductus, forefoot abductus, external malleolar torsion, external tibial torsion, external femoral torsion, tight lateral hamstrings.

○   **List the radiographic angles and measurements used in the evaluation of pes valgus?**

Calcaneal inclination angle, talar declination angle, 1st metatarsal declination angle, cuboid declination angle, cuboid abduction angle, talonavicular congruency, talocalcaneal angle, cyma line position.

○   **What are the goals of therapy (Surgical or conservative) in the treatment of flatfoot.**

Relief from pain, biomechanical control of excessive pronation, prevention of progression of the deformity.

○   **Name the varus-producing osteotomies performed in the calcaneus for flatfoot correction?**

Gleich, Dwyer, Silver, Koutsogiannis.

○   **Examination of a patient in relaxed stance reveals marked abduction of the forefoot and midfoot on the rearfoot with an apparent lateral break at the calcaneocuboid joint. Medially, a significant talar bulge is seen. What plane is dominant for this deformity based on the above findings?**

Transverse plane.

O **Nonweightbearing examination of a patient with pes valgus reveals that the amount of calcaneal eversion is far greater than calcaneal abduction and midfoot abduction. On weightbearing, there is an excessive valgus position of the heel. What is the dominant plane of deformity in the patient?**

Frontal plane.

O **Posterior calcaneal osteotomies are most useful in the correction of flatfoot with what dominant plane of deformity?**

Frontal plane dominant.

O **Where is the osteotomy and bone grafting performed for the Selakovich procedure?**

Sustentaculum tali.

O **In what type of patient is the arthroereisis procedure usually performed?**

Patients who have not yet reached skeletal maturity.

O **What are some causes of congenital flatfoot?**

Vertical talus, tarsal coalitions, Z-compensated met adductus, Short Achilles tendon, hypermobility.

O **What are the indications for a rearfoot arthrodesis in a pes valgus foot?**

Severe DJD, Severe triplane deformity with pain, Paralytic deformity, and long standing rupture of TP with collapse of the foot and adaptive change.

O **What are the primary and secondary goals of surgical treatment for a pes valgus?**

Primary goal is restoration of joint stability; secondary goal is restoration of the height of the arch.

O **What are two problems with doing an isolated subtalar fusion in the correction of a severe pes valgus deformity?**

Fusion of one portion of the subtalar joint-midtarsal joint complex results in degenerative arthrosis of the other joints, and no correction occurs in the forefoot with this procedure.

O **Describe the cyma line in a pes valgus foot?**

Anterior break in the midtarsal cyma line.

O **What is Kite's angle?**

Talocalcaneal angle.

O **What is planal dominance?**

Determining via clinical and radiographic findings, the primary plane (direction of motion) of deformity and compensation – useful in determining appropriate treatment of deformity.

❍   **What is an adjunctive procedure that is most often a part of surgery for the pes valgus foot type?**

Correction of equinus element.

❍   **What is the most common cause of peroneal spastic flatfoot?**

Tarsal coalition.

❍   **What joint(s) is/are fused in the Miller procedure?**

Navicular-1st cuneiform joint and cuneiform-1st metatarsal joint.

❍   **For arthroereisis to be effective, what must be reducible?**

Heel valgus as well as forefoot varus or supinatus.

❍   **What plane of deformity does the Evans procedure predominantly corrects?**

Transverse plane.

❍   **Which procedure elevates the posterior facet by insertion of a lateral bone graft beneath it?**

Baker-Hill.

❍   **Which procedure used for flatfoot correction lengthens the lateral column of the foot?**

Evans.

❍   **Which flatfoot procedure(s) include(s) a talonavicular arthrodesis?**

Lowman procedure, subtalar arthrodesis, and triple arthrodesis.

❍   **What special radiographic views would be helpful in evaluating a patient with a pes valgus deformity?**

A stress DF lateral view (charger view), Harris and Beath views, Neutral position WB DP and Lateral views.

❍   **What do the above views accomplish?**

Stress DF lateral view used to determine if an osseous block is present at the ankle joint, HB views helpful in ruling out talocalcaneal coalition of the posterior and middle facets, Neutral position DP and Lateral views give clinician a better idea what the foot would look like in its corrected position following surgical correction as well as being helpful for unmasking metatarsus adductus in a Z-foot or compensated metatarsus adductus.

❍   **When is subtalar joint arthroereisis indicated?**

When conservative treatment is inadequate to control pathological subtalar joint pronation in flexible pes valgus deformity.

❍   **What neural structures may be encountered when performing the Evans procedure?**

Sural nerve and intermediate dorsal cutaneous nerve.

○   **When performing a triple arthrodesis for the pes valgus foot, describe the desired position of the heel and foot.**

Slight heel valgus, approximately 15 degrees of abduction of the foot from the line of progression, and a rectus forefoot-to-rearfoot relationship.

○   **When the subtalar joint is pronated, what tendons/muscles have less than optimal function?**

Peroneus longus and tibialis posterior muscles.

○   **Which calcaneal osteotomies follow the arthroereisis principle?**

Extra-articular calcaneal osteotomies (i.e. Chambers, Selakovich, Baker-Hill).

○   **Which calcaneal osteotomy uses a bone graft under the sinus tarsi to block translocation of the talus on the calcaneus?**

Chambers.

○   **Which procedure is described as a displacement osteotomy of the calcaneus shifting the posterior fragment medially until it lies below the sustentaculum tali?**

Koutsogiannis.

○   **Which procedure(s) in the correction of flatfoot includes naviculocuneiform arthrodesis?**

Miller (navicular-1st cuneiform joint fusion), Hoke (navicular-1st,2nd cuneiform fusion).

○   **Which rearfoot arthrodesis provides stability to the rearfoot and midfoot and allows for triplane correction?**

Triple arthrodesis.

○   **When performing the Evans procedure, what tendons must be retracted inferiorly?**

Peroneals.

○   **With abnormal pronation of the STJ and unlocking of the MTJ, hypermobility and loss of stability occur distally. Describe these.**

Arch fatigue and cramping from ineffective attempt of intrinsic and extrinsic muscles to recreate stability, 1st ray instability (in transverse plane get bunion, in sagittal plane get hallux limitus), contracted digits, medial distribution of body weight adding to subluxing and deforming forces.

○   **Radiographic evaluation reveals an increased DP talocalcaneal angle, an increased cuboid abduction angle, a decreased forefoot adductus angle, and decreased percentage of talonavicular congruency. What is the dominant plane of deformity in this flatfoot?**

Transverse plane.

GRAFTING

○ **How are the relaxed skin tension lines oriented on the plantar aspect of the foot?**

Transversely.

○ **What is the orientation of collagen fibers in scar tissue?**

Parallel to the longitudinal axis.

○ **Name the two organisms that are particularly destructive to skin grafts.**

Streptococcus pyogenes and Pseudomonas pyocanea

○ **Give the thickness of the various split thickness skin grafts.**

Thin = 0.008 - 0.012 inches.
Intermediate = 0.012 - 0.016 inches.
Thick = 0.016 - 0.020 inches.

○ **Name the three stages of skin graft healing.**

Plasmatic, inosculation, reorganization / reinnervation.

○ **What is the most common complication following a skin graft procedure?**

Formation of seroma / hematoma.

○ **Name three techniques for preventing seroma formation.**

Pie crusting, meshing, compressive dressing.

○ **Name the two general types of flaps.**

Random (cutaneous) and axial pattern (arterial).

○ **Name the flap designed to provide coverage of rhomboid defects without creating secondary defect.**

Limberg flap.

○ **Name the nontoxic dye used intravenously to assess viability of skin flaps.**

Fluorescein.

○ **What is the most common cause of skin flap failure?**

Vascular embarrassment.

❍ **Describe the orientation of the longitudinal axis of the elliptical incision utilized for derotating a varus 5th toe.**

Distal-medial to proximal-lateral.

❍ **How much increase in length will result from a Z-plasty made with 60 degree cuts?**

75% increase in length.

❍ **How much increase in length will result from a Z-plasty made with 30 degree cuts?**

25% increase in length.

❍ **Name the suture utilized at the apical portions of incisions that does not penetrate the epidermis of the apex, thereby, decreasing vascular damage.**

Gillie's stitch.

❍ **What should the length to width ratio be in a cutaneous (random) flap?**

One to one (1:1).

❍ **What is the minimum angle of the flap tip angle in a Z-plasty?**

35 degrees.

❍ **What is the amount of inoculum required to cause an infection?**

10 to the fifth bacteria per gram of tissue.

❍ **Name the three processes by which soft tissue wounds heal.**

Connective tissue deposition.
Epithelialization.
Contraction.

❍ **What is the process by which skin grafts must heal when placed over avascular areas?**

Bridging (vascular supply from surrounding tissue).

❍ **What is a method used to expand the graft to allow it to cover a much greater surface area?**

Meshing.

❍ **Name three methods for controlling hemostasis at the donor site.**

Ligation or cauterization of vessels.
Epinephrine soaked gauze.
Topical thrombin.

❍ **How long after skin grafting will the graft begin to "pink up"?**

Approximately 48 hours after grafting - inosculation is now taking place providing the graft with its new blood supply.

○ **What is the length to width ratio required when removing a semielliptical portion of skin?**

3:1 (This allows primary closure of the remaining wound without much tension on the skin).

○ **Name the flap that includes skin and subcutaneous tissue, but does contain muscle.**

Fasciocutaneous flap.

○ **How does one relieve tension from the bases of a flap after performing an advancement flap?**

Cutting Burow's triangles.

○ **What is the best suturing technique for areas of high tension?**

Mattress sutures.

○ **Name four indications for skin plasties.**

Skin lengthening.
Reducing redundant skin.
Redirection of old scars.
Derotation of digits.

○ **Who originally described bone morphogenic protein?**

Urist in 1965.

○ **What is the process by which freeze-dried bone reduces its antigenicity?**

Lyophilization.

○ **What is the most common complication of bone grafting?**

Failure of the graft to heal.

○ **What are the two primary causes of bone graft failure?**

Inadequate mechanical stabilization and inappropriate selection of graft material.

○ **What type of graft should be used in an avascular nonunion?**

Autogenous bone.

○ **What is the term applied to a living bone graft taken from the same species?**

Allograft.

○ **What is the term applied to a dead bone graft taken from the same species?**

Alloimplant.

○   **What are the principle functions of a bone graft?**

Osteogenesis.
Stabilization.
Replacement.

○   **While the primary advantage of cortical bone is stability, what is the primary advantage of cancellous bone?**

Facilitates osteogenesis.

○   **Define the following terms:**

Osteogenesis: transfer of viable osteoprogenitor cells causing new bone growth.
Osteoinduction: recruitment of undifferentiated mesenchymal cells by bone morphogenic.
Protein osteoconduction: "creeping substitution" of new bone as a result of ingrowth of new vessels. The graft
Serves as a scaffold for new bone to be laid down.

○   **Name the four criteria that every bone graft material should possess.**

Immunologically acceptable.
Provide osteogenesis (actively or passively).
Provide support.
Have the ability to be replaced by bone.

○   **What type of graft is coralline hydroxyapatite?**

Xenograft.

○   **Increased oxygen tension favors bone healing. What does a decreased oxygen tension promote?**

Cartilage formation instead of bone.

○   **Large (> 6cm) osseous defects are best treated by what special type of bone graft?**

Vascularized bone transfer.

○   **How much of their initial strength will cortical grafts lose secondary to osteoclastic activity?**

30-40%.

○   **Name the two major disadvantages of autogenous bone grafting.**

Limited quantity and donor site morbidity.

○   **What is the term applied to a combination of two types of bone graft material (i.e. autogenous cancellous bone and allogenic cortical bone)?**

Composite graft.

○   **Give two examples of preventing fracture or stress risers when creating a cortical window for bone grafting.**

Outlining the window with drill holes.
Using a power saw versus an osteotome.

❍ **What is the rate at which cutting cones advance during bone healing?**

50-80 micrometers per day.

❍ **How long after cancellous bone grafting does vascularization take?**

Hours after grafting.

❍ **How long after cortical bone grafting does vascularization take?**

After the 6th day.

❍ **Name the three prerequisites for bone graft healing.**

Mechanical stability.
Vascularization of the graft bed.
Close contact between the graft and its host.

HALLUX ABDUCTO VALGUS

○ **What views should be included in the radiographic evaluation of a bunion deformity?**

AP (DP), Lateral, Forefoot (plantar) Axial to allow visualization of the sesamoid articulations and the crista, and an oblique if further visualization of the articular surfaces is necessary to evaluate for degenerative changes, bone stock and a dorsomedial bunion. Whenever possible, views should be weight bearing.

○ **What are the angular and positional relationships commonly measured on radiographs prior to correcting a bunion deformity?**

Hallux abductus angle (HA, normal less than 15 degrees).
Intermetatarsal angle (IM, normal less than 8-12 degrees).
Metatarsus Adductus angle (MA, normal less than 15 degrees).
Proximal Articular Set angle (PASA, normal less than 8 degrees).
Distal Articular Set angle (DASA, normal less than 8 degrees).
Hallux Abductus Interphalangeus (HAI, normal less than 10 degrees).
Metatarsal Protrusion Distance (MPD, + 2mm to – 2mm).
Tibial Sesamoid Position (TSP, normal is position number 3 or less).

○ **What is the relationship between the IM angle and the metatarsus adductus angle?**

As the metatarsus adductus angle increases above 15 degrees, the IM angle becomes more significant at a lower angle. A simple formula which helps demonstrate this concept is: Effective IM angle = Metatarsus Adductus angle – 15 degrees + the measured IM angle. In other words, every degree of MA angle over 15 degrees is added to the IM angle.

○ **Relative to the examination of the 1st metatarsophalangeal joint, what is meant by the term "tracking"? What is its significance?**

"Tracking" refers to the tendency for the hallux to drift back into an uncorrected position, when putting it through a range of dorsiflexion and plantarflexion, after having first placed it into a "corrected" or sagittal plane position. This tendency to drift back into an abducted position is either due to tight lateral soft tissue structures in the 1st interspace, or due to an adapted or laterally deviated articular surface of the 1st metatarsal head.

○ **What is "hallux purchase"?**

Hallux purchase is the ability of the hallux to rest firmly on the supporting surface without any attempt by the patient to actively hold it there.

○ **What is the difference between a positional deformity and a structural deformity?**

When PASA + DASA = HA angle, the deformity is considered to be structural. When PASA + DASA < HA angle, the deformity is considered to be positional or to have a positional component if the PASA or DASA are not normal.

○ **What are the preoperative indications for a Silver bunionectomy?**

A Silver bunionectomy is a partial ostectomy of the medial aspect of the 1st metatarsal head, simply a "bumpectomy." It is indicated for a patient with a large medial eminence only. In reality however, it is sometimes used as a partial measure for an elderly patient who cannot or does not want a complete correction of their bunion deformity but only relief of bump pain. In these cases, the patient should always be advised that the remainder of their deformity will continue to exist and may progress.

○   **What are the possible causes of an iatrogenic hallux varus?**

Staking the 1st metatarsal head, removing too much bone plantarly when resecting the medial eminence, fibular sesamoidectomy, vertical lateral capsulotomy, over aggressive capsulorrhaphy, over aggressive correction of the IM angle; most often several of these mistakes must be made in order to develop a hallux varus.

○   **What are the contraindications to an adductor transfer?**

The adductor tendon should not be transferred if the fibular sesamoid is degenerated, if the plantar metatarsal head articular surface is degenerated, if the fibular sesamoid is hypertrophied, or if the adductor tendon itself is atrophied.

○   **What are the uses of an adductor tendon transfer?**

To reposition the sesamoids if it is sutured into the medial 1st metatarsophalangeal joint capsule, or to reduce the intermetatarsal angle if it is sutured into the 1st metatarsal itself.

○   **What pathology is associated with a tibial sesamoid position of ≤ #4?**

Medial and dorsal shift of the 1st metatarsal. The flexor plate and the sesamoids are displaced laterally with the abduction of the proximal phalanx of the hallux. The medial capsular ligaments are stretched while the lateral capsular ligaments are contracted. An imbalance develops between the abductor hallucis muscle and the adductor hallucis muscle in which the adductor gains a mechanical advantage in its pull on the hallux. The flexor hallucis longus tendon is displaced laterally. Additionally, there may be erosion of the crista by the drifting tibial sesamoid. The tibial sesamoid may come to lie on the lateral plantar aspect of the 1st metatarsal head while the fibular sesamoid shifts into the interspace.

○   **How is metatarsus primus elevatus demonstrated on a lateral weight bearing radiograph?**

By comparing the dorsal cortical lines of the 1st and 2nd metatarsal shafts. The cortex of the 1st metatarsal will be seen to diverge from that of the 2nd metatarsal.

○   **Does an increased hallux interphalangeus affect the function of the 1st metatarsophalangeal joint?**

This deformity does not affect function directly. However, the surgeon must be vigilant not to over correct the hallux abductus due to the false impression that adequate correction has not been attained in the face of increased hallux interphalangeus.

○   **What is the most common reason for a poor post operative range of motion, even when the correct procedure is performed carefully?**

Capsular adhesions against the 1st metatarsal head.

○   **How can the chance of aseptic necrosis be reduced when performing a distal metaphyseal osteotomy such as an Austin bunionectomy?**

By preservation of soft tissue attachments to the capital fragment of the osteotomy, the periosteal blood supply is maintained.

○   **What is the correct way to resect the medial eminence? And why?**

The eminence is resected in line with the medial cortex of the shaft of the 1st metatarsal. Do not use the sagittal groove as a guide. Take care to remove more bone dorsally than plantarly. The medial plantar shelf of bone is preserved to prevent medial subluxation of the tibial sesamoid and possible development of hallux varus.

❍   **What structures are cut when excising a fibular sesamoid?**

Lateral joint capsule, fibular sesamoidal ligament, lateral head of flexor hallucis brevis, ligament between fibular sesamoid and the proximal phalanx, intersesamoidal ligament.

❍   **What is the technique for removing the fibular sesamoid?**

A linear, transverse incision is made on the lateral aspect of the 1st metatarsophalangeal joint capsule just superior to the adductor tendon and fibular sesamoid. The #15 blade is then inserted under the sesamoid and is moved proximally, taking care to stay in contact with the sesamoid as you move the blade. At the proximal aspect of the sesamoid the blade in turned 90º upward and the lateral head of the flexor hallucis brevis is severed. The blade is then re-inserted under the sesamoid and in a similar manner, the cutting edge is moved distally. When the distal aspect of the fibular sesamoid is reached, the blade is again turned 90º upward and the ligamentous attachment between the sesamoid and the proximal phalanx is severed. The sesamoid is now pulled distally and laterally while the blade is re-inserted under the sesamoid. The intersesamoidal ligament is now severed by approaching it from the proximal aspect as the sesamoid is pulled distally and laterally. The sesamoid is then removed from the surgical site and the long flexor tendon is inspected to be sure it was not severed in the process. The dissection of the sesamoid is facilitated by the use of a soft tissue tag, which can be held with a Brown Adson forceps. This tag is created with the first linear incision in the lateral capsule superior to the sesamoid. The small piece of capsule inferior to this incision, and attached to the dorsal lateral aspect of the sesamoid, is the tag.

❍   **What are the advantages of distal metaphyseal osteotomy type bunionectomies?**

The cancellous bone of the metaphysis has a better blood supply and allows for good healing; the patient is able to remain ambulatory post operatively; the procedures can be performed in a child with an open epiphysis since the epiphysis is at the base of the 1st metatarsal.

❍   **Which distal metaphyseal osteotomy type bunionectomies can correct for an abnormal PASA?**

Bicorrectional Austin; Reverdin (and its modifications), Roux, Hohmann.

❍   **What is the apical axis guide or axis guide pin and what is its purpose?**

This is a K-wire (0.045 inch), which is inserted into the metatarsal head to define the apex of the osteotomy distally. The K-wire is driven across the metatarsal head from medial to lateral and serves to align the orientation of the osteotomy cuts.

❍   **How can the axis guide pin be oriented in the frontal plane? For what purpose?**

Pin inserted from dorsal medial to plantar lateral – metatarsal head is plantarflexed as it is transposed laterally. Pin inserted from plantar medial to dorsal lateral – metatarsal head is dorsiflexed as it is transposed laterally.

❍   **How can the axis guide pin be oriented in the transverse plane? For what purpose?**

Pin inserted from distal medial to proximal lateral – the metatarsal is shortened as it is transposed laterally. Pin inserted from proximal medially to distal laterally - the metatarsal is lengthened as it is transposed laterally.

❍   **What is the potential problem with making the apex too distal when performing an Austin bunionectomy?**

Could result in fracture of the metatarsal head upon inpaction of the osteotomy.

❍   **What is the potential problem with making the osteotomy cuts too proximal when performing an Austin bunionectomy?**

This increases the lever arm for displacement of the osteotomy with weight bearing; it also places the osteotomy in diaphyseal bone, which will delay healing and lead to secondary bone callus.

○   **Does an Austin bunionectomy correct the abnormal intermetatarsal angle?**

No, it corrects relative intermetatarsal angle by moving the 1ˢᵗ metatarsal head closer to the second metatarsal head. Correcting the actual intermetatarsal angle requires moving the shaft and head of the 1ˢᵗ metatarsal closer to the second.

○   **Modifying an Austin bunionectomy to allow fixation with a dorsal cortical screw requires changing the angle between the arms of the osteotomy. How is it changed?**

The angle is reduced from approximately 60 degrees to 50-55 degrees. This allows a long dorsal arm which can be fixated with a dorsal screw.

○   **What is the Green modification to a Reverdin bunionectomy?**

The Green modification is a plantar cut which serves to protect the sesamoids. An initial plantar cut is made, which corresponds to the horizontal arm of an "L". This cut is parallel to the weight bearing surface of the 1ˢᵗ metatarsal and extends from an area approximately 1 cm. proximal to the articular surface and runs proximally, exiting the metatarsal where the head and shaft meet. This is a complete osteotomy from medial to lateral. This cut serves to protect the dorsal articular surface of the sesamoids as well as the plantar articular surface of the metatarsal head. The dorsal arm of the "L" is then created.

○   **What is the Laird modification to a Reverdin-Laird bunionectomy?**

This is when the hinge of the osteotomy is purposely fractured (cut through) and the capital fragment is transposed laterally in order to reduce the relative IM angle.

○   **What is a "geode" in reference to a bunion deformity?**

A "geode" is a degenerative cyst usually seen in the medial eminence.

○   **In what specific circumstances would a Mitchell bunionectomy be performed?**

A Mitchell is used to correct a moderately increased intermetatarsal angle in a patient with a long 1ˢᵗ metatarsal.

○   **In what specific circumstances would a Roux bunionectomy be performed?**

A Roux is used to correct a moderately increased intermetatarsal angle, and an increased PASA in a patient with a long 1ˢᵗ metatarsal.

○   **What are the indications for a Proximal Akin osteotomy?**

This osteotomy is used to correct an increased DASA.

○   **What are the indications for a Distal Akin osteotomy?**

This osteotomy is used to correct an increased hallux abductus interphalangeus.

○   **What is a "cheater" Akin osteotomy?**

This is a proximal phalangeal osteotomy (Akin) which is performed in an attempt to correct hallux abductus when the DASA and the Hallux Interphalangeus Abductus angle are normal. As such, a "cheater Akin" falls outside of the normal criteria for an Akin osteotomy.

○ What is the major indication for a Keller bunionectomy?

Painful degenerative joint disease of the 1st metatarsophalangeal joint.

○ What are the common post operative complications associated with a Keller bunionectomy?

Retraction of the hallux; lack of hallux toe purchase; instability and decreased weight bearing of the 1st MPJ; increased weight bearing of the lesser MPJ's, sometimes associated with lesser metatarsalgia and stress fractures of the lesser metatarsals.

○ What is a Juvara procedure?

An abductory, oblique closing base wedge osteotomy of the 1st metatarsal (apex medial, base lateral).

○ What are the modifications to a Juvara bunionectomy?

There are basically three modifications to a Juvara; Type A, Type B, and Type C.

Type A: standard oblique abductory base wedge osteotomy only.

Type B: the medial cortex (the hinge) is purposely cut through after the abductory wedge is accomplished and the screw is applied. This is done to allow the distal segment of the metatarsal to be plantarflexed. After the plantarflexion is accomplished, the screw is again tightened. The screw must be placed perpendicular to the long axis of the shaft to allow for plantarflexion. A second screw is then applied perpendicular to the osteotomy.

Type C: an oblique abductory base osteotomy without a wedge. The hinge, or medial cortex, is purposely cut through after the screw is applied loosely. This is done to allow the distal segment of the metatarsal to be plantarflexed. After the plantarflexion is accomplished, the screw is again tightened. The screw must be placed perpendicular to the long axis of the shaft to allow for plantarflexion. A second screw is then applied perpendicular to the osteotomy.

○ How is the screw placed, if a base osteotomy of the 1st metatarsal is fixated with a single screw?

The screw is placed halfway between the perpendicular to the long axis of the shaft of the metatarsal and the perpendicular to the osteotomy. This is a compromise. Perpendicular to the osteotomy would provide the best compression but would not prevent axial movement well. Perpendicular to the long axis of the shaft, prevents axial movement but provides poor compression.

○ What is the "Tangential Angle to the Second (metatarsal) Axis" (TASA)?

This is the angle formed by a line representing the effective articular surface of the 1st metatarsal, and the perpendicular to the longitudinal axis of the second metatarsal. The normal value is ± 5°. TASA = PASA – IM angle. TASA reflects changes in both the proximal articular set angle and the intermetatarsal angle in any given foot.

○ Name the common mid-diaphyseal osteotomies.

Ludloff osteotomy, Mau osteotomy, Scarf osteotomy.

○   **Describe a Ludloff osteotomy?**

This is a diaphyseal osteotomy extending from dorsal proximal to distal plantar.

○   **Describe the Mau osteotomy?**

This is a diaphyseal osteotomy extending from dorsal distal to plantar proximal.

○   **Describe the SCARF osteotomy.**

This is a horizontally directed (medial to lateral) Z-displacement osteotomy of the head and shaft of the 1st metatarsal. The distal arm exits the head and the proximal arm exits the shaft just distal to the base. The central limb is placed at the level of the middle and lower one third of the metatarsal shaft.

○   **What is the major complication, when transposing the distal segment of these osteotomies laterally?**

Troughing is seen if lateral displacement exceeds the cortical margins in the diaphyseal region of the metatarsal. This can result in delayed healing and in frontal plane rotation of the capital fragment.

○   **What is the name associated with an opening abductory base wedge osteotomy?**

In 1923 Trethowan performed this osteotomy, utilizing the medial eminence to keep the wedge open. In 1957 Stamm used the Trethowan technique but utilized the excised base of the proximal phalanx as the bone graft.

○   **Why is the opening abductory base wedge osteotomy a good procedure for correction of metatarsus primus adductus when it is combined with a joint destructive procedure to correct a degenerative 1st metatarsophalangeal joint?**

It is useful because it adds length to the first metatarsal and may therefore decrease the chances of post Keller metatarsalgia.

○   **Why is a staple a good choice to fixate an opening wedge osteotomy?**

It will hold open the osteotomy to the correct position even if the graft is resorbed faster than bone is laid down.

○   **What are the indications for a Lapidus procedure?**

Juvenile hallux valgus with obliquity or hypermobility at the 1st metatarsal cuneiform joint, paralytic hallux valgus, osteoarthritis, traumatic DJD secondary to an old Lisfranc injury, severe adult hallux valgus with intermetatarsal angles exceeding 18°, and as an ancillary procedure for the correction of flatfoot.

○   **What is the incidence of nonunion following a Lapidus procedure?**

In up to 10% of cases according to Clark and in 6 of 54 cases according to Saffo et al.

○   **What precautions must be taken during the soft tissue dissection for a Lapidus procedure?**

Care must be taken to preserve the medial dorsal cutaneous nerve, the attachment of the tibialis anterior, as well as the distal attachments of the posterior tibial tendon in some instances.

○   **What is the procedure first described by Loison and Balasescu?**

A closing abductory base wedge osteotomy of the 1st metatarsal in which the osteotomy is perpendicular to the shaft of the metatarsal.

O **When is the crescentic or arcuate base osteotomy a potentially useful procedure to consider?**

When the surgeon is dealing with a short metatarsal (metatarsal protrusion distance shorter than (-) 2mm. A wedge of bone is not removed thus <u>less</u> shortening is obtained.

O **Why is the crescentic or arcuate osteotomy utilized so infrequently?**

It is an inherently unstable osteotomy because there is no point of fixation, such as a hinge, and because it is technically difficult to fixate well.

O **What is the name associated with a double osteotomy of the 1st metatarsal?**

Logroscino.

O What is a Logroscino procedure?

An abductory wedge osteotomy at the base of the 1st metatarsal, either opening or closing, and a distal adductory wedge osteotomy of the 1st metatarsal head.

O **What is the major complication of any 1st metatarsal base osteotomy?**

1st metatarsal elevatus is the major complication, although shortening can also be a problem. Both may result in lesser metatarsalgia, transfer lesions, stress fractures of the lesser metatarsals, and decrease propulsive force in toe off.

O **When arthrodesing the 1st metatarsophalangeal joint, should the adductor tendon be released?**

No, when the proximal phalanx is fused to the 1st metatarsal head, the adductor tendon is no longer a deforming force and in fact it gains mechanical advantage and helps to pull the proximal phalanx and 1st metatarsal closer to the 2nd metatarsal. If the adductor is released it may cause a splaying of the forefoot and lead to a hallux varus.

O **What are the indications for a 1st metatarsophalangeal arthrodesis?**

Severe hallux valgus, hallux rigidus, Rheumatoid arthritis, salvage of failed bunion surgery, failure of Keller procedure, post infection arthrosis, post traumatic arthrosis, neuromuscular disease.

O **What is the ideal position of the hallux when arthrodesing the 1st MPJ?**

Most authors agree that the hallux should be placed in:
  Transverse plane: 15° - 25° of abductus and in line with the lesser toes.
  Frontal plane: no frontal plane rotation of the hallux.
  Sagittal plane: 10° of dorsiflexion of the hallux above the horizontal plane. This
  is a 25° angle between the hallux and the metatarsal declination angle.

O **What is a cheilectomy?**

This is a conservative procedure for hallux limitus in which the osseous proliferation found overlying the joint is excised. It is easily performed, reduces dorsal enlargement, allows increased joint motion in many cases, allows immediate ambulation, and creates minimal postoperative disability.

O   **Describe the Kessel & Bonney procedure.**

This is a procedure to address a hallux limitus deformity, in which a dorsal wedge osteotomy is performed on the base of the proximal phalanx of the hallux, to bring it into a more dorsal position. This allows the limited joint motion to occur in a more dorsal manner.

O   **What is a Regnauld procedure?**

This is a procedure in which one third of the base of the proximal phalanx is resected, removed from the surgical site, fashioned into a hemi implant configuration, and then reinserted back into the proximal phalanx as an autogenic bone graft. Sometimes referred to as the enclavement procedure. This allows for preservation of the joint while also shortening the proximal phalanx, which reduces the internal cubic content of the joint and "loosens it up".

O   **Describe a Waterman procedure.**

This is a procedure to address a hallux limitus deformity, in which a dorsal wedge osteotomy is performed on the head of the 1st metatarsal. The plantar cartilage is thus directed more dorsally which brings the hallux more dorsally.

O   **What is the Youngswick modification of the Austin bunionectomy?**

A modification of the Austin bunionectomy, which produces shortening of the 1st metatarsal and limited plantar displacement of the capital fragment. This is done by making a second dorsal cut parallel to the dorsal arm of the osteotomy but proximal to it. In this way, a small segment of bone is removed dorsally, allowing for the shortening and plantarflexion.

O   **What is the difference between hallux limitus, hallux equinus, and dorsal bunion?**

There is none. They all describe the same condition.

O   **List the common etiologies of hallux limitus.**

Metatarsus primus elevatus secondary to abnormal pronation and hypermobility of the 1st ray. Dorsiflexed position of the 1st metatarsal secondary to muscle imbalance. Dorsiflexed 1st metatarsal secondary to sagittal plane structural malalignment of the 1st metatarsal. Abnormally long 1st metatarsal. Prolonged 1st MPJ immobilization. Arthritic conditions of the 1st MPJ. Iatrogenic secondary to previous foot surgery.

O   **What is the Engel angle? How is it measured?**

This is a, so-called, simplified measurement of metatarsus adductus. It is the angle formed by the intersection of the longitudinal bisection of the second metatarsal and the longitudinal bisection of the 2nd or intermediate cuneiform.

O   **What is the relationship of the Engel angle to the metatarsus adductus angle?**

The Engel angle is generally about 3° higher than the traditional metatarsus adductus angle.

O   **A patient presents to your office complaining of a painful deformed hallux. Pertinent radiographic measurements include PASA 8 degrees, DASA 6 degrees, HAIA (hallux interphalangeus) 20 degrees, IMA 8 degrees. What is the BEST procedure to address this patients painful deformity?**

Distal Akin procedure.

O   **Which surgical procedure would be most appropriate to correct a PASA of 12 degrees and an IM angle of 7 degrees?**

Reverdin procedure.

HEEL PAIN

❍ **Rupture of the Achilles tendon with in the elderly population will most often occur at what location?**

The insertion into the calcaneus.

❍ **Distally, the plantar fascia INITIALLY inserts into which of the following anatomical structures?**

The superficial transverse metatarsal ligament or natatory ligament.

❍ **Upon examination of a lateral weight bearing x-ray of the foot an inferior heel spur would most often be found with in?**

The origin of the FDB.

❍ **How will a symptomatic Haglund's Deformity present clinically?**

Pain upon palpation of the posterior superior lateral aspect of the calcaneus.

❍ **Is a plantar fasciotomy an advisable treatment alternative for a heel spur syndrome of one month in duration?**

NO! Recent onset plantar fasciitis and/or heel spur syndrome respond well to conservative treatment options including cortisone injections, heel cord and plantar fascia stretching, strapping, orthoses, physical therapy modalities, night splints, and casting.

❍ **Is heel spur syndrome/plantar fasciitis commonly seen in the adolescent population?**

NO! This is generally an adult problem.

❍ **Describe the clinical presentation of retrocalcaneal bursitis.**

Pain on palpation of both sides of the achilles tendon with observable erythema and edema without pain on ankle range of motion and having a negative bone scan.

❍ **Fat pad degeneration of the heel will present clinically as?**

Plantar central heel pain on palpation in geriatric patients.

❍ **Entrapment of the first branch of the lateral plantar nerve is theorized to be an etiology of?**

Heel spur syndrome.

❍ **The first branch of the lateral plantar nerve is referred to as ?**

Baxter's nerve.

❍ **The windlass mechanism was described by?**

Hicks.

❍   **What type of stress is imposed upon the plantar fascia during weight bearing?**

Tension stress.

❍   **Degenerative tears within the Achilles tendon are characterized by healing with what type of tissue?**

Adipose.

❍   **A contracted Achilles tendon would result in what type of ankle deformity?**

Equinus.

❍   **Where does the lateral band of the plantar fascia insert?**

It inserts into the styloid process of the base of the 5th metatarsal.

❍   **How does one make the diagnosis of calcaneal apophysitis in a 14-year-old boy?**

Subjective pain elicited by medial and lateral compression of the calcaneus.

❍   **What is the average length of the Achilles tendon in the adult population?**

15cm.

❍   **The blood supply to the Achilles tendon is decreased at a point approximately ___cm above its insertion on the calcaneus.**

4 to 5

❍   **Are corticosteroid injections around the Achilles tendon recommended?**

They are not recommended because of the risk of rupture.

❍   **In most cases of acute Achilles tendinitis or tendinosis without rupture, the initial treatment approach should be?**

Ice massage, heel lift, stretching exercises, rest and NSAIDs.

❍   **The tibial nerve divides at he level of the medial malleolus into superficial and deep branches; the superficial branch, which runs subcutaneously above, the laciniate ligament is named?**

The medial calcaneal nerve.

❍   **Which nerve supplies sensory innervation to the medial and plantar heel pad?**

Medial calcaneal.

❍   **What are the possible points of entrapment of the first branch of the lateral plantar nerve (to the abductor digiti quinti)?**

The first point occurs on its course to the abductor digiti quinti muscle. It is compressed by the deep fascia of the abductor hallucis muscle and the medial head of the quadratus plantae muscle. The next point is where the nerve crosses just distal to the medial calcaneal tuberosity in the vicinity of the heel spur. Here it may be compressed against the bone and ligaments.

○ **Pain elicited upon medial-lateral compression of the calcaneus, should make one suspicious of?**

Calcaneal stress fracture.

○ **Pain which is located inferior to the central heel, proximal to the site of plantar fasciitis, and which does not radiate, is most likely to be?**

Heel pad atrophy or inferior calcaneal bursitis.

○ **Barring injuries, the differential diagnosis for inferior calcaneal heel pain should include?**

Plantar fasciitis/heel spur syndrome, inferior calcaneal bursitis, heel pad atrophy, nerve entrapment (posterior tibial, medial calcaneal, 1st branch of lateral plantar nerve), seronegative spondyloarthropathies, rheumatoid arthritis, gout, pseudogout, sarcoidosis, thyroid abnormalities, Paget's disease, and infections.

○ **What is the bursal projection?**

This is the posterior superior projection of the calcaneus.

○ **Is the retrocalcaneal bursa an anatomic bursa or an adventitial bursa? Where is it?**

It is an anatomic bursa, its presence is consistent. It is located in the recess between the bursal projection and the anterior margin of the Achilles tendon. It extends 2 mm below the bursal projection.

○ **What is the retroachilles or pretendon or Achilles bursa? Where is it?**

This is an adventitial bursa which forms over the posterior superior calcaneus, between the skin and the bone/tendon due to friction and pressure from the shoe counter. This is the predominant finding in a "pump bump".

○ **What is the Phillip-Fowler angle? Its significance?**

The Phillip-Fowler angle is a measurement used to determine the presence of a Haglund's deformity. It is the angle formed by the intersection of a line along the posterior calcaneus and a line along the inferior calcaneus. The normal value is 44-69 degrees. Any angle over 75 degrees is said to be suggestive of a Haglund's deformity and cause painful symptoms.

○ **What is the "total angle" of Ruch described in 1974? Its significance?**

This is the combination of the Phillip-Fowler angle + the calcaneal inclination angle. Normal is less than 90 degrees. This angle takes the calcaneal inclination into consideration. As the inclination increases, the posterior superior calcaneus becomes more prominent and likely to cause a problem.

○ **What are "parallel pitch lines?" Their significance?**

A line is drawn along the inferior calcaneus (as in a calcaneal inclination angle). A perpendicular to this line is then drawn from the posterior margin of the posterior facet of the STJ. A third line is then drawn parallel to the inferior calcaneal line, at the top of the second line. If the bursal projection lies above this third line, then a significant Haglund's deformity is said to exist.

○ **How is Achilles tendinosis defined radiographically?**

On a lateral nonweightbearing radiograph, greater than 9 mm of thickening of the Achilles tendon, at a point 2 mm superior to the bursal projection.

○ **Describe the clinical presentation of a patient with a posterior calcaneal heel spur.**

These patients generally have localized pain to palpation directly over the bony prominence. There may be pain with dorsiflexion of the foot.

INFECTIONS

○ **What is the causative organism for Pitted Keratolysis?**

Corynebacteria.

○ **What color does pitted keratolysis fluoresce when examined with a Wood's lamp?**

Coral red.

○ **What is the most common infecting organism in superficial white onychomycosis?**

Trichophyton mentagrophytes.

○ **Which disease is characterized by weeping granulomas and sinus tracts of the foot due to infection with Pseudoescheria boydii.**

Madura foot.

○ **What is the treatment for cutanea larva migrans?**

Topical thiabendazole.

○ **Name a highly contagious form of scabies seen in patients with HIV disease.**

Norwegian scabies.

○ **A Cub Scout complains of a prickly sensation on his legs after wading in a lake on a sunny day in November. His scout troop is visiting a wildlife preserve in Upstate New York. Red macules appear hours later, which begin to itch over the remainder of the evening. Diagnosis?**

Cercarial dermatitis (swimmer's itch).

○ **What is the causative organism for hand, foot, and mouth disease?**

Coxsackie virus (most commonly A16).

○ **A 16 year old boy presents with asymptomatic umbilicated papules on the dorsum of his right foot. Most likely diagnosis?**

Molluscum contagiosum.

○ **What medication is used to treat chromoblastomycosis?**

Itraconazole.

○ **What is the most common causative organism for septic arthritis?**

Staphylococcus aureus.

○   **What is the correct dosage regimen for treating a serious diabetic infection of the foot with IV Trovafloxacin?**

200 mg q 24 hours.

○   **What antibiotic is contraindicated in patients with a seizure history?**

Imipenam/cilastin.

○   **What consultation is important when placing a patient on IV aminoglycosides?**

Audiology.

○   **The most common infecting organism in pediatric septic arthritis is Staphylococcus aureus. What organism is also very prevalent?**

Kingella kingae.

○   **Which oral antifungal is known to cause bony malformations and CNS defects in the fetus when administered to pregnant females?**

Fluconazole.

○   **Which oral antifungal is known to cause taste disturbances and green vision?**

Terbinafine.

○   **Identify 2 oral antimicrobials that may incite serious adverse effects in those patients currently taking an HMG CoA reductase inhibitor?**

Itraconazole and Erythromycin.

○   **What malignancy can develop in an area of chronic osteomyelitis?**

Epidermoid carcinoma.

○   **What is Brodie's abscess?**

A metaphyseal bone abscess surrounded by granulation tissue and sclerotic bone in cases of chronic osteomyelitis.

○   **What organism is usually responsible for erysipelas?**

Group A Streptococcus.

○   **What cultures might one order to diagnose an extrapulmonary tuberculosis infection of a pedal phalanx?**

Acid fast cultures.

○   **In what type infection is eosinophilia classically observed?**

Parasitic infections.

○   **What titers are drawn to aid in the diagnosis of rheumatic fever?**

Anti-streptolysin O titers.

○   **What antigens are present on the cell membrane of Staphylococcus that may be of diagnostic benefit when cultures are unattainable?**

Teichoic acids.

○   **For which disease are Osler's nodes and Janeway lesions of diagnostic benefit?**

Infectious endocarditis.

○   **If choosing an antibiotic for prevention of infectious endocarditis in a high risk individual, what treatment approach should be followed when the patient is already on an antibiotic for some other reason?**

Choose an antibiotic from a different class.

○   **What is the name of the skin lesion at the site of the tick bite in Lyme Disease patients?**

Erythema chronicum migrans.

○   **Which antibiotic is known to turn body fluids an orange color?**

Rifampin.

○   **Which antibiotic has been implicated as a cause of tendon ruptures?**

Ciprofloxacin.

○   **Which antibiotics should only be used with extreme caution in diabetic patients on oral sulfonylureas?**

Sulfonamides.

○   **Why is Ceftin (cefuroxime) contraindicated in pregnant patients?**

Chance of renal tubular lesion formation in the fetus and mother.

○   **What skin manifestation is characteristically seen in 2-6% of patients with sepsis secondary to Pseudomonas aeruginosa?**

Ecthyma gangrenosum.

○   **In which genetic disease is infection with Pseudomonas aeruginosa a common problem?**

Cystic fibrosis.

○   **What nail disease is caused by Pseudomonas aeruginosa?**

Green Nail Syndrome.

○   **Which infection characteristically gives a fruity odor?**

Infections with Pseudomonas aeruginosa.

○ **What topical medication should be used for infected burn wounds when heavy eschar is present?**

Mafenide (Sulfamylon).

○ **A patient presents with dystrophic nails that have flecks of pigmentation throughout the nail plate. For which pathogen is this suggestive as a cause of onychomycosis?**

Aspergillus niger.

○ **According to the Cierny and Mader classification for osteomyelitis, what would the designation be for an HIV positive patient with diffuse osteomyelitis of the right calcaneus?**

Stage 4 Bs.

○ **In what instance are fluoroquinolones a possible risk for the induction of seizures?**

Concomitant administration of NSAIDs and a fluoroquinolone may increase penetration of drug into CSF and interact with excitatory neurotransmitters.

○ **Ciprofloxacin and Itraconazole may be subject to specific drug interactions due to their metabolism. Explain.**

These drugs are inhibitors of the hepatic cytochrome p450 enzyme pathway.

○ **Which microorganism is responsible for Lyme Disease?**

Borrelia burgdorferi.

○ **What skin test is often positive in patients with septic arthritis caused by Mycobacterium tuberculosis?**

PPD.

○ **A 55 year old female gardener steps on a rose bush lying on the ground. A thorn penetrates the 1st MPJ. What organism must be considered as a possible etiology for her painful, swollen septic joint?**

Sporothrix schenckii.

○ **What are 2 white blood cell labeled bone scans?**

Indium 111 and Tc HMPAO.

○ **Which group of organisms is not covered by Clindamycin?**

Gram negative aerobes.

○ **Which group of organisms is not covered by Levofloxacin?**

Anaerobes.

○ **Name 2 antibiotics that can be used to treat pseudomembranous colitis.**

Metronidazole and oral Vancomycin.

O   **Which cephalosporin is often used in place of ceftriaxone (Rocephin) due to its similar coverage and cost efficiency?**

Cefotaxime (Claforan).

O   **What organism is the major concern in patients with lymphangitis and cellulitis of the lower extremity?**

Beta Hemolytic Streptococcus.

O   **What bacteria are often infecting organisms secondary to trauma associated with salt water injury?**

Vibrio species.

O   **In which type puncture wound of the foot might you see Eikinella corrodens on culture results?**

Toothpick wounds (used).

O   **What mold has been documented as a cause of a life-threatening sepsis following pedal infection in immunocompromised patients, particularly those who garden in their bare feet?**

Fusarium.

O   **How is cutanea larva migrans transmitted to humans?**

Contact with hookworm-infested dog or cat feces on public beaches.

O   **What lower extremity manifestations may present in a person with Neiserrial meningitis?**

Palpable purpura on the lower legs.

O   **What color do mycobacteria appear against a dark background on acid-fast stains?**

Yellow or red.

O   **What are the typical symptoms of a patient with pseudomembranous colitis?**

Watery diarrhea, fever, and cramping.

O   **Why are antidiarrheals contraindicated in cases of pseudomembranous colitis?**

Life-threatening toxic megacolon may result.

O   **What arthritic disorder of the feet, ankles, and sacroiliac joints is associated with bacterial infection (e.g. Chlamydia)?**

Reiter's Syndrome.

O   **What dermatologic manifestation is seen on initial presentation of patients with Rocky Mountain Spotted Fever?**

Erythematous macules on the ankles and wrists.

○   **Name 3 causes of Steven-Johnson Syndrome.**

Herpesvirus infections I, pregnancy, drugs.

○   **In what infectious disease does one observe the classic "strawberry tongue."**

Scarlet fever.

○   **Which antibiotic is contraindicated in children under eight years of age due to its potential to cause permanent discoloration of the teeth?**

Tetracycline.

○   **For what infection are multinucleated giant cells on Tzanck smear diagnostic?**

Herpes infections.

○   **With which class of antibiotics does potential major adverse effects exist in patients taking Digoxin?**

Macrolides.

○   **With which oral antifungal have potential serious adverse effects been documented with patients taking tricyclic antidepressants?**

Terbinafine.

○   **Patients with sickle cell anemia, and other hemoglobinopathies, have a higher incidence of osteomyelitis with which organism?**

Salmonella.

○   **What does gas in the soft tissues indicate?**

An anaerobic infection. Aerobic metabolism does not produce gas.

○   **Is "saline aspiration" from the leading edge of cellulitis a useful clinical tool?**

No, it is rarely productive for pathogens.

○   **What are the classic signs of a necrotizing infection?**

Blistering and necrosis but these are generally late findings.

○   **What is a clue to early diagnosis of a necrotizing infection?**

The patient's marked systemic toxicity in light of what appears to be "ordinary" cellulitis.

○   **What is another name for clostridial myonecrosis?**

Gas gangrene.

JUVENILE HALLUX ABDUCTO VALGUS

O **What percent of adult patients with HAV deformity is a result of untreated juvenile HAV?**

Approximately 40% of adults with HAV have evidence of the deformity before the age of 20.

O **Is there a gender predisposition towards juvenile HAV?**

Before age of 14 the male: Female prevalence of HAV is approximately 1:1.
However, in adolescents greater than age 14, the deformity was found to be three times more common in females.

O **Explain why a child with Spastic Cerebral Palsy often develops juvenile HAV.**

Scissor gait due to tight posterior muscles, including the triceps surae produce an equinus force at the ankle joint. The joints distally try to compensate and dorsiflex the foot via pronation throughout the majority of contact phase of gait. The flexible pronated foot does not provide an effective lever for the muscles and tendons that are needed to stabilize the first ray during propulsion.

O **What musculoskeletal deformity usually accompanies juvenile HAV in the absence of extrinsic and systemic etiologies?**

Metatarsus adductus.

O **What systemic disease results in a high incidence of juvenile HAV?**

Juvenile rheumatoid arthritis.

O **Name the pedal factors that are implicated in causing the severity of juvenile HAV deformity.**

Round metatarsal head, atavistic cuneiform, hypermobile first ray, hyperpronation, a high intermetatarsal angle.

O **Why are the failure rates for soft-tissue bunionectomy procedures so high?**

Soft tissue procedures do not correct the osseous deformity.

O **When planning surgical intervention, when is the appropriate time?**

Surgical intervention is safely performed after the closure of the epiphysis.

O **What are the indications for surgery prior to closure of the epiphysis?**

Progressive deformity, uncontrollable deforming forces, rigid metatarsal head adaptation, pain, and severe deformity.

O **What are the principles in juvenile HAV surgery?**

Restore joint alignment, reduce intermetatarsal angle, plantargrade first ray, address etiology of deformity, post operative control of deforming forces.

○   **Concerning juvenile HAV, what are the indications for performing a Lapidus procedure.**

Severe increased intermetatarsal angle with instability of the first ray usually associated with neuromuscular and collagen disorders.

○   **The only indication for epiphysiodesis in juvenile HAV surgery is?**

Increased intermetatarsal angle.

○   **Describe two techniques for performing epiphysiodesis.**

Lateral stapling of the growth plate or insertion of bone graft.

○   **The most common complication of epiphysiodesis is?**

Recurrence.

○   **Name two procedures for juvenile HAV that address the atavistic cuneiform.**

Fowler and Lapidus.

○   **Name all types of internal fixation that are acceptable to use across a growth plate.**

Smooth K-wires.

○   **The basal metatarsal osteotomy is employed to?**

Reduce the severe intermetatarsal angle.

○   **The metatarsal head osteotomy may be employed to correct?**

Mild increased intermetatarsal angle, as well as to restore joint congruity (PASA) and relocate the sesamoids.

○   **At what age does the epiphysis appear radiographically?**

Approximately 2 years of age.

○   **At what age do the sesamoids begin to ossify?**

10-12 years of age.

○   **What is the major difference regarding the ossification of the lesser metatarsals and the first metatarsal?**

The first metatarsal epiphysis is at the base, compared to the head of the lesser metatarsals.

○   **The adductor tendon transfer is used as an adjunctive procedure to?**

Relocate and maintain the corrected sesamoid position.

○   **The Hiss procedure is?**

A transfer of the abductor hallucis to the dorsomedial proximal phalanx of the hallux.

O **Is there a strong familial predilection for juvenile HAV?**

Yes, literature reports vary between 50 - 78% familial incidence.

O **What is the most common postoperative complication for the closing base wedge osteotomy?**

Elevatus.

O **Regarding juvenile HAV, phalangeal osteotomies are indicated for?**

Phalangeal osteotomies, such as the Akin, should only be used when there is a structural abnormality within the proximal phalanx.

MEDICAL LAW

○ **What entity issues an indictment? Is the accused present?**

An indictment is issued by a grand jury with the accused absent.

○ **A license to practice Podiatric Medicine is issued by?**

The State Medical Board or a similar administrative agency of state government.

○ **"Due Process of Law" prevents the revocation of a podiatrist's license without?**

The law requires a "hearing after notice."

○ **If a patient presents himself for examination and treatment, but does not discuss payment terms with the doctor, is the doctor entitled to payment?**

Yes they are, on the theory of "implied contract."

○ **When a hospital denies staff privileges to a doctor, what are the doctor's legal rights?**

He is entitled to an impartial hearing, which is reviewable by a court.

○ **What is the difference between a "claims made" malpractice insurance policy and an "occurrence" malpractice policy?**

With an "occurrence" policy, as long as policy <u>was in force</u> at the time that an alleged malpractice occurred, then the coverage is provided, even if the policy is no longer in force. With a "claims made" policy, the insurance policy must be in force at the time that a malpractice claim is filed. For instance, if a doctor has a "claims made policy" in force in 1999 but drops the insurance when he retires in the year 2000. Then, in 2000 a malpractice claim is filed against him for an alleged malpractice which occurred in 1999. He is not covered for this incident because his insurance was not in force in 2000 when the claim is made.

○ **What are the obligations of a doctor to his insurance carrier?**

The doctor is obligated to notify the carrier promptly when he receives a claim; to cooperate with the adjuster and lawyer in preparing his defense; to appear at trial if requested; and to submit to depositions before trial.

○ **Under what general category is a medical malpractice case (based on negligence)?**

Tort.

○ **What is a tort?**

A private wrong not based on contract.

○ **What is an injunction?**

A court order to do or to refrain from doing a specific act.

○   **When are punitive damages awarded?**

Only where intentional torts are involved. In some states, punitive damages are awarded, only for wanton, willful, and malicious behavior.

○   **A malpractice case will not be tried before a jury unless?**

Either party demands a jury.

○   **When may a civil malpractice case be tried in a United States District Court?**

When the parties to the case are citizens of different states and the matter in question is over $75,000.00.

○   **On whom, is the burden of proof in a civil malpractice case?**

On the plaintiff, by a preponderance of the evidence.

○   **Under what rule, may a doctor be responsible for his nurse's negligence?**

Under the rule of "respondeat superior."

○   **What is the primary function of an expert witness?**

To render an opinion regarding proximate causation and regarding the standard of care.

○   **What is the degree of care required of a podiatrist?**

The national standard of care; that degree of care which is defined by the ordinary standard of care.

○   **Is a doctor who exercises the utmost care, but gets a bad result, liable?**

He is liable only if he promised or guaranteed a result, which was not achieved.

○   **Will getting a patient's informed consent protect the doctor against a claim of battery?**

Yes.

○   **What are the elements of medical malpractice?**

There must be: a) a duty b) a breach of the duty c) damage d) a causal relationship between the breach of duty and the damage (proximate cause).

○   **What is the term, used to describe the selection and questioning of jurors?**

Voir Dire.

○   **What is the rule of "stare decisis?"**

The rule that a court tends to follow its previous decision based on similar facts.

○   **What is the burden of proof in a malpractice case?**

The plaintiff must prove his case by a preponderance of the evidence.

○ **What is an assault?**

A threat of physical harm.

○ **What is slander?**

A false, malicious, spoken, publicized statement may be the basis of a slander claim.

○ **Can punitive damages be awarded in a successful suit for slander?**

Yes.

○ **What is the first document filed in court in a malpractice case.**

The complaint.

○ **During the process of "voir dire", how may prospective jurors be challenged?**

Jurors may be challenged for cause or peremptorily.

○ **How is a contract formed?**

A contract comes into being when an offer is made by one party, accepted by another party, and consideration passes between them. A contract may be either implied or express.

○ **How is the doctor-patient relationship usually established?**

By implied contract, without verbally expressed terms.

○ **Which Medicare coverage is supplemental?**

Medicare Part B, for which the policyholder pays a premium.

○ **When is Worker's Compensation not paid?**

When the accident arises outside the scope of employment.

○ **What is the difference between a crime and a tort?**

Crimes are violations of statute or ordinance and are offenses against the government or public. A tort is a private wrong not based on contract.

○ **What is an "express contract?"**

An express contract is an actual agreement between the parties, the terms of which are openly stated in distinct and explicit language, either orally or in writing.

○ **According to the Controlled Substances regulations, what are the classifications of controlled substances?**

Classification of Substances
    Schedule I - high potential for abuse, no currently accepted medical use lack of accepted safety.

Schedule II - high potential for abuse, currently accepted medical use, abuse may cause severely psychological or physical dependence.
Schedule III - high potential for abuse, currently accepted medical use, abuse may cause severe psychological or physical dependence.
Schedule IV- low potential for abuse, currently accepted medical use, abuse may cause limited dependence.
Schedule V- same as IV but to lower degree.

○ **Narcotics prescribed by podiatrists for use in clinical practice are which Schedule?**

Schedule II.

○ **What is a doctor's recourse when he is owed money by a patient who files for bankruptcy?**

The doctor may file a claim in bankruptcy court and may receive all or part of the amount owed, or nothing depending on the circumstances of the case.

○ **What is Medicaid?**

A joint Federal-State program to aid the poor, aged, blind, disabled - the "Medically Needy."

○ **When is a "Covenant Not To Compete" valid?**

When it is reasonable as to duration and geographic extent.

○ **The governmental power to regulate the practice of Podiatric Medicine is derived from what power of the state?**

The state's police power.

○ **Is residence in a state a requirement to get a license to practice podiatric medicine in that state?**

No it is not.

○ **True or False. It is a crime not to report suspected elder abuse to authorities.**

True.

○ **In a malpractice case based on negligence, what types of damages are awarded?**

Compensatory damages and possibly loss of consortium.

○ **If you treat a patient at the scene of an accident, can you be liable?**

You are not liable as long as no compensation was paid to you or expected by you and your actions were made in a good faith effort to help.

○ **What is defamation?**

Defamation of character occurs when one person communicates to a second person about a third in such a manner that the reputation of the person about whom the discussion was held is harmed.

○ **What is libel?**

A written defamatory statement.

○ **What is slander?**

Spoken defamation is termed slander.

○ **What may a non-expert witness testify about?**

Generally, facts only, not opinion.

○ **Can a doctor shelter his assets from a malpractice claimant, after a claim is filed, by transferring his assets?**

No, he may be subject to both civil and criminal liability.

○ **What is the generic term for civil wrongs other than breach of contract?**

Torts.

○ **Can damages in a battery case include punitive damages?**

Yes they can.

○ **What is the Statute of Limitations? Is it the same in every state?**

The Statute of Limitations is the time period in which a patient has to file a malpractice suit. This is <u>not</u> the same in every state.

○ **Under what circumstances may the statute of limitations be extended?**

It may be extended where patient is a minor; where doctor is out of state; and where doctor conceals patient's true condition or patient did not promptly discover true condition.

○ **What is the definition of a minor?**

A minor is any person under the age of majority. A minor is incapable of giving effective consent for the administration of medical treatment. Depending on state law, the age of majority may be eighteen or twenty-one. Exceptions are made in medical emergencies and for mature and emancipated minors.

○ **How should a doctor terminate his or her care of a patient before the completion of care?**

Termination should be with a written notice sent by certified mail and should explain the patient's medical problem. The patient must be afforded the opportunity to acquire the needed services from another physician.

○ **In terms of the litigation process, what is discovery?**

This is the heart of civil litigation, including medical malpractice. This is the process by which each side learns the pertinent facts of the opponent's case. The purpose is to allow each party to test the other party's facts and determine the strength of the other party's case.

○ **What is an interrogatory?**

An interrogatory is a technique of discovery in which one party responds, under oath, to written questions submitted by the other party.

○   **What is a deposition?**

A deposition is a technique of discovery in which oral examination, including cross-examination, under oath, of witnesses and parties is performed.

○   **What is a subpoena duces tecum?**

A technique of discovery; subpoena duces tecum is a court order requiring production of books and records for examination by the other party.

○   **In terms of the litigation process, what is a motion?**

A motion is a document filed with the court in which the moving party asks the court to take some action.

○   **What is a motion of summary judgment?**

A common motion, in medical malpractice litigation, in which the party, usually the defendant, asks the court to decide the case based on the law only as there is no dispute concerning the facts.

○   **What is the doctrine of res ipsa loquitur?**

A technique in which the plaintiff tries to show a breach of the standard of care without direct evidence.
Res ipsa loquitur (the thing speaks for itself) is a device by which the plaintiff may be able to prove, through circumstantial evidence, that a particular defendant breached the standard of care. For example, a forceps in found in a patient's abdomen after a surgery.

MEDICINE

○ **What are the signs and symptoms of hyperthyroidism?**

Signs: Fever, tachycardia, wide pulse pressure, CHF, shock, thyromegaly, tremor, liver tenderness, jaundice, stare, hyperkinesis, and pretibial myxedema. Mental status changes include somnolence, obtundation, coma, or psychosis.

Symptoms: Weight loss, palpitations, dyspnea, edema, chest pain, nervousness, weakness, tremor, psychosis, diarrhea, hyperdefecation, abdominal pain, myalgias, and disorientation.

○ **Describe Leriche's syndrome?**

Impotence with buttock, calf, and back pain. It usually occurs with aortoiliac disease.

○ **Where is the most common site of peripheral aneurysms that develop in the lower extremity from arteriosclerosis?**

The popliteal artery.

○ **Define a hypertensive emergency.**

Elevated diastolic blood pressure > 115 mm Hg with associated end organ dysfunction or damage.

○ **Livedo reticularis commonly develops on what body parts?**

The legs. Livedo reticularis is a bluish red discoloration of the skin resulting from vasospasm of the arterioles. This condition is worsened by exposure to cold.

○ **What is Virchow's triad?**

1) Injury to the endothelium of the vessels.
2) Hypercoagulable state.
3) Stasis.

○ **What does normal ventilation with decreased lung perfusion suggest?**

Pulmonary embolism.

○ **What are the most common signs and symptoms of PE?**

Tachypnea (92%), CP (88%), dyspnea (84%), anxiety (59%), tachycardia (44%), fever (43%), DVT (32%), hypotension (25%), and syncope (13%).

○ **What test is considered the gold standard for the diagnosis of DVT? For the diagnosis of PE?**

1) DVT: venography; duplex scanning is rapidly becoming the new standard.
2) PE: pulmonary angiography.

○ Atelectasis accounts for what percentage of postoperative fevers?

90%.

○   **Why do we care about postoperative atelectasis?**

If it persists for more than 72 hours, pneumonia may develop. Perioperative mortality rates are then 20%. Incentive spirometry is an important therapy for the prevention of atelectasis.

○   **What is the risk of placing a patient with COPD on high flow O$_2$?**

Suppression of the hypoxic ventilatory drive.

○   **What is the anticoagulant treatment schedule for a PE?**

IV heparin until PTT is 2 to 2.5 times normal. After a day, warfarin is added until the INR is greater than 2.0. If clots recur, consider a Greenfield filter in the IVC. Pulmonary embolectomy is only necessary in cases of massive embolisms.

○   **Sarcoidosis is most common I what race and age group?**

African Americans between 20 and 40 years of age.

○   **What are the side effects of INH treatment for TB?**

Neuropathy, pyridoxine loss, lupus-like syndrome, anion-gap acidosis and hepatitis.

○   **What are the classic signs and symptoms of TB?**

Night sweats, fever, weight loss, malaise, cough, and a greenish yellow sputum most commonly observed in the mornings.

○   **A young man with atraumatic back pain, eye trouble, and painful red lumps on his shins develops bloody diarrhea. What is the point of this question?**

To remind you of the extraintestinal manifestations of inflammatory bowel disease, such as ankylosing spondylitis, uveitis, and erythema nodosum, not to mention kidney stones.

○   **What is the defining characteristic for obesity?**

A weight 20% above the height/weight recommendation.

○   **What are the major causes of pancreatitis?**

Alcohol and biliary tract disease.

○   **What principle hormone protects the human body from hypoglycemia?**

Glucagon.

○   **What are the two primary causes of primary adrenal insufficiency?**

Tuberculosis and autoimmune destruction. Together, they account for 90% of cases.

○   **What is the most common cause of hyperphosphatemia?**

Acute and chronic renal failure.

○   **What are the signs and symptoms of primary adrenal insufficiency?**

Fatigue, weakness, weight loss, anorexia, hyperpigmentation, nausea, vomiting, abdominal pain, diarrhea, and orthostatic hypotension.

○   **What is the most common cause of hypoglycemia seen in the Emergency Department?**

An insulin reaction in a diabetic patient.

○   **What signs and symptoms are helpful for diagnosing thyroid storm?**

Eye signs of Graves' disease, a history of hyperthyroidism, widened pulse pressure, hypertension, a palpable goiter, tachycardia, fever, diaphoresis, increased CNS activity, emotional lability, heart failure, and coma.

○   **What is the most common cause of secondary adrenal insufficiency and adrenal crisis?**

Iatrogenic adrenal suppression from prolonged steroid use. Rapid withdrawal of steroids may lead to collapse and death.

○   **How long must a generalized tonic-clonic seizure last without a period of consciousness to be considered status epilepticus?**

30 minutes. Status epilepticus may result from grand mal seizures or anticonvulsant therapy withdrawal.

○   **What factors may precipitate migraine headaches?**

Bright lights, cheese, hot dogs and other foods containing tyramine or nitrates, menstruation, monosodium glutamate and stress.

○   **A 26 year old woman complains of a throbbing, dull, unilateral headache that last for hours then goes away with sleep. She also has been nauseated and has vomited twice. She reports small areas of visual loss plus strange zigzag lines in her vision. What is the diagnosis?**

Classic migraine headache. Classic migraine accounts for only 1% of migraines. It can be differentiated from the common migraine because it involves visual disturbances of scotomata and fortification spectra, in addition to all the other migraine symptoms.

○   **Which type of headache usually afflicts adults?**

Tension headaches. This is a bilateral "bandlike" fronto-occipital headache accompanied by constant pain. Tension headaches are generally muscular in nature therefore a patient may also have tense neck and scalp muscles.

○   **A resting tremor is usually related to what disease?**

Parkinson's disease. Parkinson's tremors are generally asymmetrical and have the characteristic "pill rolling" appearance.

○   **Pseudohypertrophy of the calves is characteristic of which type of muscular dystrophy?**

Duchenne's muscular dystrophy. Hypertrophy is caused by fatty infiltration of the muscles.

❍   **What is the most common presenting symptom of multiple sclerosis (MS)?**

Optic neuritis (about 25%)

❍   **What is the most common cause of syncope?**

Vasovagal or simple fainting (50%)

❍   **What is the toxic dose of naloxone?**

None. Narcan is a safe drug and may be given in large quantities. The usual adult dosage is 0.4 - 2 mg IV; the usual pediatric dose is 0.01 mg/kg. Narcan may precipitate acute withdrawal and may therefore be titrated to effect.

❍   **What drug is the most common pharmaceutical cause of true allergic reactions?**

Penicillin. It accounts for approximately 90% of true allergic drug reactions and more than 95% of fatal anaphylactic drug reactions. Parentally-administered penicillin is more than twice as likely to cause a fatal anaphylactic reaction as compared to orally-administered penicillin.

❍   **After penicillin, what is the most common cause of anaphylaxis-related deaths?**

Insect stings. Approximately 100 deaths occur in the US annually because of anaphylaxis induced by insect stings.

❍   **Are the nodules of erythema nodosum more often symmetrical or asymmetrical in distribution?**

Symmetrical. These nodules are distinctive, bilateral, tender nodules with underlying red or purple shiny patches of skin that develop in a symmetrical distribution along the shins, arms, thighs, calves, and buttocks.

❍   **Is there an effective treatment for erythema nodosum?**

No. The disease usually lasts several weeks, but the pain associated with the tender lesions can be relieved with non-steroidal anti-inflammatory agents.

❍   **What is Lhermitte sign in ankylosing spondylitis?**

A sensation of electric shock that radiates down the back when the neck is flexed. This is a sign that atlantoaxial subluxation and C-spine instability may be present.

❍   **What other diseases may produce Lhermitte sign?**

Rheumatoid arthritis and multiple sclerosis.

❍   **A patient on chronic steroids presents with weakness, depression, fatigue, and postural dizziness. What pathological process should be suspected? What is the treatment?**

Adrenal insufficiency. The treatment is to administer large "stress doses" of steroids.

❍   **If adrenal insufficiency is suspected, what test should be performed? What drug should be prescribed?**

A serum cortisol level should be drawn before administering a large dose of steroids. Dexamethasone is the preferred agent because it will not interfere with subsequent tests if they are needed.

○ **What cardiac complication commonly occurs with SLE, juvenile rheumatoid arthritis, and rheumatoid arthritis?**

Pericarditis.

○ **How should a new monoarthritis be approached in a patient with rheumatoid arthritis?**

Assume it is septic until proven otherwise. The risk for infection is higher in a joint that has been previously injured for affected by arthritis.

○ **What painful bone abnormality often complicates steroid therapy in patients with rheumatoid arthritis or systemic lupus erythematosus?**

Avascular necrosis of the femoral head, femoral condyles, or bones of the foot.

○ **What disease produces erythematous plaques with dusky centers and red borders resembling bull's eye targets?**

Erythema multiforme. This disease can also produce non-pruritic urticarial lesions, petechiae, vesicles, and bullae.

○ **What can cause erythema multiforme?**

Viral or bacterial infections, drugs of nearly all classes, and malignancy.

○ **What spinal lesion can produce shin splints?**

Compromise of the L5 and S1 nerve roots. This lesion may also produce calf pain that mimics the symptoms of deep vein thrombosis.

○ **A patient with back pain who cannot walk on his or her toes has a lesion at which level?**

S1.

○ **A patient with back pain who cannot walk on his or her heels has a lesion at which level?**

L5.

○ **What is the most common cause of chronic renal failure?**

NIDDM.

○ **Below what platelet count is spontaneous hemorrhage likely to occur?**

$< 10,000/mm^3$.

○ **How can an overdose of warfarin be treated? What are the advantages and disadvantages of each treatment?**

Fresh frozen plasma (FFP) or Vitamin K. However, if there are no signs of bleeding, temporary discontinuation may be all that is necessary. Treatment depends on the severity of symptoms, not the degree of prolongation of the prothrombin time.

○ **What is the only coagulation factor not synthesized by hepatocytes?**

Factor VIII.

○ **Which four hemostatic alterations are seen in patients with liver disease?**

Decreased protein synthesis leading to coagulation factor deficiency.
Thrombocytopenia.
Increased fibrinolysis.
Vitamin K deficiency.

○ **What is von Willebrand's disease?**

An autosomal dominant disorder of platelet function. It causes bleeding from mucous membranes, menorrhagia, and increased bleeding from wounds. Patients with von Willebrand's disease have less (or dysfunctional) von Willebrand's factor.

Von Willebrand's factor is a plasma protein secreted by endothelial cells and serves 2 functions: (1) It is required for platelets to adhere to collagen at the site of vascular injury which is the initial step in forming a hemostatic plug. (2) It forms complexes in plasma with factor VIII which are required to maintain normal factor VIII levels.

○ **When using Doppler, what audible characteristics differentiate arterial from venous flow?**

Arterial flow is characterized by sharp, brisk changes in pitch throughout the cardiac cycle (higher pitched during peak systole and lower pitched during diastole; also termed multiphasic). Venous flow varies with the respiratory cycle and venous signals are lower pitched and more consistent throughout the cardiac cycle (monophasic).

○ **What is the diagnostic test of choice for documenting DVT?**

Duplex scan (ultrasound). The accuracy of physical examination for DVT is generally quoted to be 50%.

○ **What are the major sequelae of untreated streptococcal infections?**

Acute glomerulonephritis unrelated to treatment and rheumatic heart disease.

○ **What substances increase PVC's?**

Caffeine, alcohol, and tobacco.

○ **What organism is commonly found in infected wounds caused by animal bites?**

Pasturella multocida. The second most common is staphylococcus aureus.

○ **What is the most common cause of secondary lymphedema?**

Malignant metastases to the lymph nodes. Lymphatic fibrosis secondary to surgery is another cause.

○ **What disorder is most likely to be confused with erythema nodosum?**

Cellulitis.

○ **Where is the most common site of thrombophlebitis?**

The deep muscles of the calves, particularly the soleus muscle.

○ **Under what conditions does trench (immersion) foot develop?**

Trench foot occurs when the extremity is exposed for several days to wet, cold conditions at temperatures that are above freezing. The extremity develops superficial damage resembling partial thickness burns.

○ **Describe pernio (chilblain).**

Exposure of an extremity for a prolonged period of time to dry, cold but above freezing temperatures. Patients develop superficial, small, painful ulcerations over the chronically exposed areas. Sensitivity of the surrounding skin, erythema, and pruritis may also develop.

○ **What is the therapy of choice to neutralize heparin in a patient who was inadvertently administered too much?**

Protamine. 1 mg of protamine will neutralize about 100 units of heparin. The maximum dose of protamine is 100 mg.

○ **Why are quinolones contraindicated for children?**

Quinolones impair cartilage growth.

○ **A patient is in anaphylactic shock. She happens to be taking B-blockers. She is not responding to epinephrine. What alternative agents might you consider?**

Norepinephrine, diphenylhydramine, and glucagons.

○ **An absent knee jerk involves which spinous level?**

L4.

○ **An absent Achilles reflex involves which spinous level?**

S1.

○ **Paresthesias of the great toe involves which spinous level?**

L5.

○ **Paresthesias of the little toe involve which spinous level?**

S1.

○ **What is the cause of erysipelas?**

Group A, B-hemolytic streptococcus.

○ **What is Brudzinski sign?**

Flexion of the neck produces flexion of the knees.

○ **What is Kernig's sign?**

Extension of the knees from the flexed thigh position results in strong passive resistance.

❍   **What are the elements of Noninvasive Vascular Studies to evaluate arterial flow?**

Ankle/Arm Index (Ischemic Index), Arterial Doppler Waveforms, Segmental Pressures, Pulse Volume Recordings, Photoplethysmograph (PPG) Waveforms.

❍   **What are the characteristics of a normal arterial waveform?**

A triphasic waveforms with rapid upstroke, large amplitude, dichrotic notch, rapid downstroke. This represents high velocity and normal volume blood flow. The faster the flow, the steeper the wave.

❍   **What is the minimal rate of flow necessary to produce and audible signal?**

4 cm/sec.

❍   **What does the dichrotic notch in the arterial Doppler represent?**

Reverse blood flow.

❍   **What is the difference between the tracing made with a unidirectional Doppler and that of a bi-directional Doppler?**

With a unidirectional Doppler, both forward and reverse flow is seen above the baseline. With a bi-directional Doppler, forward flow is above the baseline and reverse flow is below the baseline.

❍   **What pressure difference between pressure cuffs is considered indicative of an occlusive lesion?**

20-30 mm Hg.

❍   **Why are ankle/arm indexes and segmental pressures considered unreliable in a diabetic patient?**

Due to the high incidence of calcified arteries (medial calcific sclerosis) which require higher pressures to occlude and therefore do not correlate to true systolic pressures.

❍   **Half of all patients with valvular disease present a definite history of what?**

Acute rheumatic fever.

❍   **How does acute rheumatic fever affect the heart? What is the mechanism.**

Sensitivity reaction to the hemolytic streptococcus which produces its damage without actually being present in the heart. During the acute phase there is pancarditis, myocarditis (Aschoff bodies) and endocarditis. Usually pancarditis and myocarditis resolve but chronic endocarditis with scarring of the valves occurs.

❍   **What is the most common heart valve affected in valvular heart disease?**

Mitral Valve.

❍   **IV drug abusers with valvular heart disease usually have which valve affected?**

Tricuspid valve.

❍   **What is the predominant causative organism for subacute bacterial endocarditis in IV drug abusers?**

Staphylococcus.

○ **A patient has paroxysmal substernal pain that is worse with exertion and relieved by rest. What is the diagnosis?**

Angina Pectoris.

○ **Describe unstable angina.**

Anginal pain that is increasing in severity, duration, and frequency.

○ **A patient is having a MI. What extra heart sound would be most commonly heard on auscultation?**

S4 or atrial gallop.

○ **What enzymes are detected in the blood after a MI? Which is seen first?**

Creatinine phosphokinase (CPK) rises and falls most rapidly. Serum glutamic oxaloacetic transaminase (SGOT) is increased within 6 to 12 hours and reaches its peak in 2 to 3 days then reverts to normal. Lactic dehydrogenase (LDH) is of greater specificity than SGOT and is elevated for a longer period.

○ Which of the cardiac enzymes seen after a MI is an index of myocardial necrosis?

LDH.

○ **What are the classic ECG findings seen in the leads overlying the infarcted cardiac muscle?**

Significant Q waves in leads ordinarily dominanted by R waves, Abnormal S-T segment elevation, and abnormal inverted T waves.

○ **What are the two types of hypertension? Which is the most common of the two types?**

Essential hypertension (unknown cause) – most common (>90%) and secondary hypertension.

○ **What is the most common reason a male patient would have iron deficiency anemia?**

GI blood loss.

○ **Hypochromia and microcytosis are morphological findings in which type of anemia?**

Iron Deficiency anemia.

○ **Which anemia can have resultant neurologic manifestations? What are the neurologic manifestations seen with this anemia?**

Anemia due to Vitamin B_{12} deficiency can cause peripheral neuropathy, posterolateral column degeneration, and behavioral changes

○ **What is polycythemia vera?**

A neoplastic myeloproliferative disorder with red cell proliferation and a variable degree of thrombocytosis and leukocytosis. (majority of symptoms due to hyperviscosity of the blood).

○   **What is Hemophilia A caused by?**

Bleeding disorder due to an inherited deficiency of factor VIII.

○   **Are males or females affected more frequently in Hemophilia A?**

Only men are clinically affected since this is a disease that is transmitted in a sex-linked recessive pattern.

○   **You suspect Hemophilia A. What blood tests will confirm this diagnosis?**

Prolonged PTT and low Factor VII coagulant activity. Bleeding time and PT will be normal.

○   **What is the deficient plasma coagulant protein in Christmas Disease?**

This is Hemophilia B and the deficiency factor is Factor IX.

○   **What is Von Willebrand's disease?**

Hereditary bleeding disorder transmitted as an autosomal dominant trait characterized by prolonged bleeding time with a normal platelet count and frequently a prolonged PTT.

○   **What platelet count would constitute thrombocytopenia?**

Less than 150,000 per ul.

○   **Risk of spontaneous and serious bleeding increases at platelet counts less than what?**

Less than 20,000 per ul.

○   **What is the most common reason for an eosinophilia?**

Parasitic infections. Also seen in acute allergic attacks, and in some chronic skin diseases i.e. pemphigus, psoriasis.

○   **What is the most common reason for a lymphocytosis?**

Viral infections.

NAIL, DIGIT, AND FOREFOOT SURGERY

○   **What are the common causes of recurrence following a phenol/alcohol procedure?**

Common causes of recurrence include: "old" or expired phenol, insufficient phenol application to affected areas; removing insufficient toenail border; inadequate hemostasis.

○   **"Granuloma pyogenicum" refers to?**

Granulation tissue in the medial or lateral nail groove.

○   **Where is the hyponychium anatomically?**

Lies under the free margin of the nail bed.

○   **How does an exostoses differ from osteochondroma?**

Fibrocartilage caps the bone instead of a hyaline cap.

○   **The advantages of the Frost procedure include?**

Maximum exposure to the nail matrix area.

○   **What are the common digital blocks utilized for anesthesia prior to a surgical nail procedure?**

Two-point block, H-block, and the unilateral block of Steinberg.

○   **Effective initial treatment for an infected ingrown toenail border is?**

Partial nail avulsion, PO antibiotic therapy, foot soaks.

○   **This patient above was effectively treated at first, then returned six months later with pain secondary to incurvation of the nail fold in the absence of erythema, edema, and purulence. What procedure is recommended?**

Partial nail avulsion with matrixectomy.

○   **What is the proper sequence of the steps used during the sequential reduction of a dorsally subluxed MPJ?**

Release of extensor hood expansion, release of collateral ligaments, release of plantar joint tissues.

○   **What are the advantages in the use of the flexor tendon transfer for digital surgery?**

Possible prevention of a joint fusion; Decreased incidence of mallet toe; Realignment of the metatarsophalangeal joint.

❍   **What is a more common reported disadvantage of the flexor tendon transfer in digital surgery?**

Prolonged edema and stiffness.

❍   **Given severe osteomyelitic destruction of a distal phalanx secondary to an ulcerated distal heloma, what procedure would be indicated?**

Distal Symes amputation.

❍   **What is the Hoffman procedure?**

Resection of metatarsal heads 1-5.

❍   **What is an advantage of the plantar transverse incisional approach for the rheumatoid forefoot reconstruction?**

The plantar approach provides good exposure to the severely plantarflexed metatarsal heads.

❍   **What is the "hood apparatus"?**

The "hood apparatus" or "extensor expansion" is the medial and lateral fibrous extensions of the extensor tendon. It is composed of tendinous contributions from the long and short extensor tendons as well as from the lumbricales and interossei. The "hood apparatus" functions such that the pull of the long and short extensor tendons creates dorsiflexion of the proximal phalanx at the metatarsophalangeal joint via the "sling" portion of the apparatus.

❍   **How many interossei muscles are there and where do they insert?**

Three plantar interossei which insert on the base of the proximal phalanx, medially and four dorsal interossei which insert on the base of the proximal phalanx laterally except the first dorsal interossei which inserts from medially. Together with the flexor digiti quinti brevis, there are eight intrinsic muscles that function as a pair for each lesser digit.

❍   **What are the forces and functions of the interossei muscles?**

The pull of the interossei muscles neutralizes the force of the flexor muscles at the metatarsophalangeal joints.

❍   **Describe the extensor substitution phenomenon as an etiology for hammertoes?**

Extensor substitution occurs during propulsion, swing phase, and heel contact when the extensor digitorum longus and brevis muscles are active. It may occur as a result of an equinus and an anterior cavus foot type and may manifest as a result of peripheral neuropathy, as the intrinsic muscles are often affected first.

❍   **What are the benefits of a compressive, post-operative forefoot bandage?**

Reduction of edema, maintaining positioning as healing occurs, and diminished risk of infection.

❍   **What is the most common etiology of the heloma molle?**

Typically the head of the proximal phalanx of the fifth digit is displaced against the lateral condyle of the base of the fourth proximal phalanx. The fourth toe may be longer or shorter than customary, altering the normal convex-to-concave relationship between toes.

❍   **Describe the pathology and correction of brachymetatarsia?**

The toe is usually straight, but in an extended position, and floats above the weight-bearing plane. A deep sulcus is present beneath the short metatarsal. Surgical treatment usually is directed toward lengthening the shortened metatarsal, often lengthening extensor tendons and skin as well.

○ **What are the disadvantages of the flexor tenotomy and capsulotomy?**

Decrease in digital purchase postoperatively, high rate of recurrence of deformity, and limited application.

○ **What may be considered the major cause for the recurrence of a hammered digit following digital surgery?**

Instability at the metatarsophalangeal joint.

○ **What is the relationship between the deep transverse intermetatarsal ligament (DTIL) and the interossei and lumbricales?**

The plantar and dorsal interossei lie dorsally and the lumbricales plantar.

○ **What is the primary cause of flexor stabilization?**

Excessive pronation causing instability.

○ **Overpowering of or by the flexor digitorum longus muscle will result in what deformity?**

Dorsiflexion of the MPJ, and plantarflexion of the PIPJ and DIPJ.

○ **To develop the classic hammertoe, the pull of which tendons are needed?**

Both the FDL and FDB are needed.

○ **The PIPJ arthrodesis effectively?**

Converts the toe to a rigid lever on which the long flexor and extensor tendons can function effectively.

○ **What are the indications for an extensor tenotomy procedure?**

Indicated in a flexible extensor hammertoe but may also effectively be used as an adjunct to the digital arthroplasty.

○ **At what level should an extensor tenotomy procedure be performed?**

Proximal to the extensor hood apparatus.

○ **What are the results of a flexor tendon transfer?**

Functions like the PIPJ arthrodesis, removes a dynamic deforming force, and stabilizes the MPJ in plantarflexion.

○ **What are the advantages of the peg-in–hole arthrodesis?**

Increased bone-to-bone contact, increasing the fusion rate. No fixation is actually required. Shortening of an elongated toe.

○ **What planes may be involved in dislocation of a metatarsophalangeal joint?**

Sagittal, transverse, and frontal may all be involved.

O   **What is the fourth-fifth intermetatarsal angle that is generally considered symptomatic and elevated?**

9 degrees or higher.

O   **What does the lateral deviation angle measure?**

It measures structural deformity of the fifth metatarsal itself.

O   **What is a logical step-wise approach to the severely overlapping fifth toe.**

Resection of the head of the proximal phalanx, lengthening of the extensor digitorum longus tendon, dorsal and medial capsulotomy, release of the plantar plate, and removal of a plantar skin wedge. K-wire stabilization may also be required.

O   **Describe the Hibbs procedure?**

The extensor digitorum longus tendons are detached distally and tenodesed into the midfoot, at the level of the third metatarsal base.

O   **What is the most commonly chronically dislocated joint in the foot?**

Second metatarsophalangeal joint.

O   **Which anatomical structure is generally considered the most significant factor in the stabilization of the MTPJ?**

Plantar plate.

O   **What is the Lachman test?**

With the second metatarsal immobilized and the proximal phalanx held in 20 to 25 degrees of dorsiflexion, the proximal phalanx is translated vertically in a dorsal direction. This is a test for MPJ instability or the ability to resist dorsal subluxation.

O   **What studies are traditionally used to assess instability at the second metatarsophalangeal joint?**

Plain radiographs, MRI, and arthrography.

O   **What is the pathophysiology of an intermetatarsal neuroma?**

Perineural fibrosis.

O   **What is the epidemiology of the intermetatarsal neuroma?**

Female predominance, unusual in persons younger than 18 year old, it is most common for a patient to have a single neuroma, rather than multiple ones, and most often found in the second or third interspaces.

O   **The intermetatarsal neuroma most often involves which nerve?**

Third common digital branch of the medial plantar nerve.

○   **What is an uncommon finding when re-operating on a Morton's neuroma?**

Inordinate scar tissue is usually NOT seen. An amputation neuroma or an intact accessory nerve trunk distal to the DTIL is seen as well as the DTIL (deep transverse intermetatarsal ligament), which has reapproximated itself.

○   **What anatomical structure(s) is cited as entrapping the intermetatarsal nerve?**

The deep transverse intermetatarsal ligament.

○   **What are the specific complications associated with surgical excision of the neuroma?**

Stump neuroma, vascular embarrassment, and digital and/or MPJ mechanical instability.

○   **Joplin's neuroma involves which anatomical structure?**

Plantar proper digital nerve.

○   **Common causes of this entrapment neuropathy known as a Joplin's neuroma include:**

Sporting activities such as running, soccer, basketball, snow skiing that involve pivoting, impact, and motion surrounding the first metatarsophalangeal joint. Chronic compression from a tight shoe. A prominent medial epicondyle of the first metatarsal.

○   **The neuroma known as Iselin's neuroma is found:**

In the 1st interspace.

○   **Hueter's neuroma is found:**

In the 4th interspace.

○   **The relaxed skin tension lines in the sub-metatarsal head region or plantar forefoot run:**

Parallel to the plantar transverse lines along the lesser digits.

○   **The incisional planning of a derotational arthroplasty of the 5th digit includes:**

2 semi-elliptical incisions coursing from proximal lateral to distal medial.

○   **What is Freiberg's Infraction?**

Osteochondrosis of the metatarsal head most commonly the second, appearing most often in the second decade of life.

○   **What is a common etiology of an epidermal inclusion cyst?**

It may follow a surgical procedure in which epidermis is introduced subepidermally, forming an intradermal foreign body that causes pain and inflammation.

○   **Which of the following describes a benign longitudinal ungual pigmentation?**

Longitudinal melanonychia.

❍   **A longitudinal ungual pigmentation in a fair skinned individual without any precursor or injury should indicate:**

Possible precursor for acral lentiginous melanoma and the need for nail avulsion and biopsy.

❍   **What is the etiology of keloids?**

Represent fibrous reactions at surgery or injury sites. The reaction involves myofibroblasts and may be related to abnormalities of capillary endothelium during granulation. Keloids may be associated with fibromatoses and with peptic ulcers and enostoses.

❍   **Does infantile digital fibromatosis require treatment?**

The lesions occur in fingers and toes and may regress spontaneously or require surgical excision.

❍   **Do digital mucous cysts communicate with the joints?**

Yes, they may communicate with the distal interphalangeal joint and will often recur with local curettage.

❍   **The clinical presentation of a child with shortened digits and hallux valgus may signify?**

Myositis ossificans progressiva.

❍   **A solitary, subungual, reddish-purple, painful lesion may be a?**

Glomus tumor.

NERVE ENTRAPMENT, NERVE COMPRESSION, AND NEUROPATHIES

❍ **Sensory nerves composed of 4 – 14 bundles of nerve fibers separated by perineurium and covered by an epineurium are known as?**

Peripheral Nerves.

❍ **The central core of a myelinated nerve fiber is known as?**

The Axon.

❍ **Myelin is deposited around the nerve cells by?**

Schwann Cells.

❍ **What is myelin?**

Lipid substance that acts as an excellent insulator.

❍ **What is myelin dependent upon for it's continued existence?**

The Schwann cell and its adjacent axon.

❍ **The group of nerves that form the basis of neuronal function in the lower extremity is known as?**

The lumbosacral plexus.

❍ **The lumbar plexus is formed by?**

The first 3 lumbar nerves, and part of the 4th lumbar nerve.

❍ **In distal axonopathies with segmental demyelinization what happens to the Schwann cells?**

The Schwann cells are preserved.

❍ **What is Saltatory Conduction?**

Nerve impulses conducted, along a myelinated nerve, from Node of Ranvier to Node of Ranvier.

❍ **What is the Node of Ranvier?**

A small uninsulated area between Schwann Cells.

❍ **What is the distance between the Nodes of Ranvier?**

Approximately 1 millimeter.

O   **What happens at the Node of Ranvier?**

Ions can flow easily between the extracellular fluid and the axon.

O   **What is the purpose of Saltatory Conduction?**

To allow myelinated nerve fibers to conduct impulses at a higher velocity than unmyelinated fibers.

O   **What happens to the nerve fiber if the cell body is destroyed at the level of the spinal cord?**

The entire nerve dies.

O   **Distal degeneration of a myelinated nerve fiber is known as?**

Wallerian degeneration.

O   **A primary loss of myelin results in:**

A significantly slower nerve conduction velocity.

O   **A nerve injury which results in a transient loss of sensation and/or function lasting from several days to several weeks is known as?**

Neuropraxia.

O   **The type of nerve injury which results in paranodal demyelinization, followed by remyelinization is known as?**

Neuropraxia.

O   **A nerve conduction velocity test for a patient with a neuropraxia would show?**

A slower nerve conduction velocity.

O   **The use of tourniquets and casts may result in which type of nerve injury?**

Neuropraxia.

O   **A crush or severe compressive nerve injury involving degeneration of the axon is known as?**

Axonotmesis.

O   **A severe nerve injury which results in initial Wallerian degeneration, then healing, is know as?**

Axonotmesis.

O   **What is the prognosis for restoration of function after axonotmesis?**

Good.

O   **What happens to nerve conduction velocity after axonotmesis heals?**

Nerve conduction velocity is usually slightly delayed.

O   **A severe nerve injury which results in permanent Wallerian degeneration and complete loss of sensation and/or function is known as?**

Neurotmesis.

O   **A nerve conduction velocity test for a patient with a neurotmesis would show?**

No nerve action potentials.

O   **Trophic changes to the skin would indicate involvement of?**

The autonomic nervous system.

O   **Pain and/or paresthesia radiating both proximal and distal upon palpation or percussion of a peripheral nerve is known as?**

Valleix's sign.

O   **Pain and/or paresthesia radiating distally upon palpation or percussion of a peripheral nerve is known as?**

Tinel's sign.

O   **Injury or compression to the medial proper digital nerve to the Hallux may also be known as?**

Joplin's neuroma.

O   **Joplin's neuroma is almost always observed in association with?**

A bunion deformity.

O   **Pain and/or numbness on the medial side of the first metatarsal and hallux is often associated with?**

Joplin's Neuroma.

O   **Swelling of a peripheral nerve due to entrapment and/or compression is known as a?**

Neuroma.

O   **Morton's neuroma is classically located in which web space?**

Third web space.

O   **A patient complaining of pain/numbness and/or burning in the metatarsal head area on the plantar foot, near the third web space is probably suffering with?**

A Morton's neuroma.

O   **Entrapment/Compression of the superficial peroneal nerve is also known as?**

Lemont's nerve injury.

❍   **Tarsal Tunnel Syndrome is due to nerve injury to which nerve(s)?**

Tibial nerve.

❍   **Which anatomic structures form the Tarsal Tunnel?**

Medial malleolus, calcaneus, and the lacinate ligament.

❍   **Excessive pronation, space occupying lesions, tenosynovitis, ganglions, edema, and fracture of the ankle, talus or calcaneus may result in?**

Tarsal Tunnel syndrome.

❍   **Burning pain of the plantar foot, numbness of the plantar foot and toes, and referred pain proximally indicates which nerve injury?**

Tarsal tunnel syndrome.

❍   **External pressure from the shoe counter may cause injury to which nerve?**

Sural nerve.

❍   **Which nerve courses around the neck of the fibula, and through the peroneus muscle belly?**

Common peroneal nerve.

❍   **Trauma or compression/entrapment of which nerve will result in weakness and/or sensory loss along the lateral aspect of the foot and leg?**

Common peroneal nerve.

❍   **Which diagnostic test would be most helpful in the diagnosis of nerve compression/entrapment?**

Nerve conduction velocity.

❍   **Destruction of nerve tissue via chemical measures is known as:**

Neurolysis.

❍   **Surgical excision of a nerve or nerve section is known as:**

Neurectomy.

❍   **Dorsal beaking at the talo-navicular or navicular-cuneiform joints may result in:**

Anterior Tarsal Tunnel Syndrome.

❍   **Trauma to the anterior ankle such as ankle sprain or ankle swelling may cause compression of?**

Anterior tibial or deep peroneal nerve.

❍   **A severe inversion ankle sprain may result in injury to?**

The superficial peroneal nerve.

❍   **Peroneal tendon pathology, lipoma or cysts, and pressure from the shoe counter may result in injury to?**

The sural nerve.

❍   **A viscous intracellular fluid which fills the axon is known as?**

Axoplasm.

❍   **When injecting corticosteroids for nerve injuries it is important to inject into or around the nerve?**

Around the nerve.

❍   **Unconscious proprioception is assessed by?**

Romberg's test.

❍   **Positioning a joint in the position most likely to compress or stretch the nerves crossing it is known as?**

Phalen's sign.

❍   **Fasciculations suggest dysfunction of?**

Lower motor neuron disease.

❍   **Hyperactive reflexes are indicative of?**

Upper motor neuron disease.

❍   **During a nerve conduction velocity test the velocity at which the larger or faster conducting fibers propagate an impulse is known as?**

Conduction velocity.

❍   **The peripheral nerve is composed of three types of components, which are?**

Sensory, motor, and autonomic.

❍   **The most common cause of peripheral neuropathy in the western world today is?**

Diabetes mellitus.

❍   **Bulbous paranodal swelling of nerves at an entrapment sites are known as?**

Tadpoles.

❍   **The surgical excision of a damaged nerve section is known as?**

Neurectomy.

❍   **Approximation of severed nerve endings is known as?**

Neurorrhaphy.

○   **Peripheral neuropathy of a single named nerve is known as?**

Mononeuropathy.

○   **Peripheral neuropathy of multiple peripheral nerves is known as?**

Polyneuropathy.

○   **Large sensory fibers transmit precisely synchronized impulses known as?**

Epicritic sensations.

○   **Small sensory fibers transmit noxious impulses known as?**

Protopathic sensations.

○   **What is the most common demyelinating disease?**

Multiple sclerosis.

○   **Pathology pertaining to the spinal nerve roots is known as?**

Radiculopathy.

○   **When a patient walks with small steps, keeping his knees semiflexed, thereby avoiding stretching the nerve root he is exhibiting a?**

Positive Neri's sign.

○   **Any difference in size greater than ½ inch in the circumference of the patient's gastrocnemius indicates?**

Atrophy of the smaller side.

○   **A positive Laségue test indicates?**

Sciatic nerve irritation.

○   **Dryness of the skin, and loss of sweating in diabetics is a sign of?**

Autonomic neuropathy.

○   **The most common form of diabetic neuropathy is?**

Distal symmetrical polyneuropathy.

○   **Genetic peripheral neuropathies may be due to?**

Inborn errors of metabolism (porphyria, amyloid), Storage disorders (leukodystrophies, Refsum's disorder), and phenotypic groups (Charcot- Marie-Tooth, Friedreich's ataxia).

○   **The peripheral nerve pathology associated with Herpes Simplex Virus is?**

Acute radiculitis usually sciatic in distribution.

❍   **The neurologic sequelae of Herpes Zoster are?**

Radiculitis, myelitis, and polyradiculoneuropathy.

❍   **Neurological symptoms associated with viral hepatitis include?**

Mononeuropathy of the sciatic and/or common peroneal nerves.

❍   **The most common neurological symptom of HIV infection is?**

Peripheral neuropathy.

❍   **The most common type of peripheral neuropathy associated with AIDS is?**

Distal symmetric polyneuropathy.

❍   **The most common neurological symptom associated with alcoholism is?**

Polyneuropathy.

NEUROMUSCULAR DISEASES

O   **What is the anatomical difference between upper motor neuron disease and lower motor neuron disease?**

Patients with upper motor neuron involvement have pathology proximal to the anterior horn cell. Lower motor neuron disease begins at the anterior horn cell and extends distally to include the peripheral nerve, neuromuscular junction, and myofibril.

O   **Describe sensation and tone in neuromuscular disease.**

In neuromuscular disease, there may or may not be sensory involvement. Tone may be normal, decreased, or increased.

O   **Describe the basic nature of upper motor neuron disease.**

The basic nature of the upper motor neuron disease involves spasticity. Patients may or may not have sensory loss. There is relatively good preservation of the soft tissues since the anterior horn cell has been preserved.

O   **Which neuromuscular disease characteristically shows mixed upper and lower motor findings.**

Amyotrophic lateral sclerosis.

O   **Describe the basic nature of lower motor neuron disease.**

Lower motor neuron disease involves flaccid paralysis. It is characterized by normal to low tone, and significant muscle wasting since the nerve supply to the muscle has been interrupted. There is also sensory loss and an absence of spasticity.

O   **Name some common causes of lower motor neuromuscular disease and their level of involvement.**

From most proximal to distal:
> Spinal cord-anterior horn cell: Poliomyelitis, Wernig-Hoffman, Spinal muscle atrophy, Spina bifida
> Peripheral Nerve: Diabetes mellitus, vitamin deficiency (B_1, B_6, B_{12} (most common)), direct trauma, Charcot Marie Tooth Disease
> Neuromuscular Junction: Myasthenia gravis, Post polio syndrome
> Muscle (Myopathy): Muscular dystrophy, polymyositis, dermatomyositis,
> Myotonic Dystrophy (adult muscular dystrophy)

O   **What is the most common muscular dystrophy in childhood and adults and how are they inherited?**

The most common muscular dystrophy in childhood is Duchenne's muscular dystrophy occurring 1 in 3500 newborn males by sex-linked inheritance. Becker's muscular dystrophy is also sex-linked and occurs in about 1 in 35,000 newborn males. On the molecular level, Duchenne's and Becker's muscular dystrophy is caused by a mutation in the dystrophin gene which codes for the dystrophin muscle protein which is normally present in the cell membrane of normal muscle. The most common muscular dystrophy in adults is Myotonic dystrophy that occurs by dominant inheritance. On the molecular level myotonic dystrophy occur as a mutation on chromosome 19 and is a duplication of the CTG repeats. In non affected individuals there are up to about 30 CTG repeats. In individuals with myotonic dystrophy the number of CTG repeats is increased dramatically.

○ **How is classic Duchenne muscular dystrophy diagnosed?**

It is initially suspected due to delayed ambulation and is always evident by school age. Laboratory testing reveals at least a 10 fold increase in serum creatinine phosphokinase (CPK). Muscle biopsy shows an absence of dystrophin, an abnormal variation of muscle cell size, and an increase in connective and fat tissue. DNA testing is available to diagnose Duchenne muscular dystrophy and shows a mutation in the dystrophin gene. The dystrophin gene is one of the largest genes which is why it is very vulnerable to mutation.

○ **How does Becker's muscular dystrophy differ from Duchenne's muscular dystrophy?**

Becker's muscular dystrophy is more benign, occurs at a later age of onset, and progresses more slowly. There is a greater than five-fold increase in CPK and patients typically do not become wheelchair bound until their teens. Patients with Becker's muscular dystrophy frequently survive into their fifth and sixth decade. However, there is no difference between Duchenne's muscular dystrophy and Becker's muscular dystrophy on muscle biopsy. Both diseases are inherited sex linked.

○ **How are the muscular dystrophies characterized?**

Low tone, proximal muscle weakness, and calf hypertrophy.

○ **How is myotonic dystrophy different from other muscular dystrophies?**

Myotonic dystrophy is characterized by distal muscular weakness and is the only muscular dystrophy that may present with a foot drop.

○ **What are some additional problems that patients with muscular dystrophies often have beside the primary muscle involvement?**

Cardiomyopathy is common in sex-linked muscular dystrophy. Endocrine abnormalities are common in myotonic dystrophy. Mental retardation is associated with muscular dystrophy.

○ **Name the 3 basic forms of myotonic dystrophy.**

The classical form is the adult onset and is characterized by myotonia and weakness of the distal muscles of the arms and legs, with ocular, and pharyngeal weakness and early onset of cataracts. There is an early childhood form with onset between ages 5 and 10 years which is characterized by myotonia, mental retardation, and generalized weakness. The most severe form of myotonic dystrophy is the congenital form which presents with severe neonatal weakness or still birth.

○ **What is the basic nature of inflammatory myopathies?**

Inflammatory myopathies present with normal to low muscle tone, and a proximal symmetrical motor weakness. Patients have muscle soreness and tenderness as well as markedly elevated CPK levels, in other words, similar presentation to muscular dystrophies.

○ **What conditions are inflammatory myopathies associated with?**

Interstitial lung disease, cardiomyopathies with arrhythmias, esophageal dysmotility, and various autoimmune syndromes.

○ **Describe the orthopedic manifestations of neurofibromatosis.**

Neurofibromatosis is a disease process characterized by café au lait spots, subcutaneous nodules and neurofibromas. There may be soft tissue hypertrophy which can involve one extremity on the entire half of the body. The most important skeletal manifestations are scoliosis and congenital pseudoarthrosis of the tibia. Frequently, the family history is positive for this disorder. Crowe's criteria are used to diagnose the condition. Two of the following should be present: (1) a positive family history, (2) a positive biopsy of a lesion, (3) a minimum of 6 café au lait spots, greater than 1.5 centimeters in diameter, or (4) multiple subcutaneous nodules

❍ **Give a general description of poliomyelitis.**

Poliomyelitis is an infection caused by Type I, Type II, or Type III poliomyelitis virus, a member of the enterovirus group. The virus gains entry into the body through the gastrointestinal or respiratory tract, causing an acute infectious process which has a special affinity for the anterior horn cells of the spinal cord as well as for the bulbar nuclei of the brain stem. Infection causes necrosis of these cells with loss of innervation to the motor units. Sensation remains intact. Widespread prophylactic vaccination has greatly reduced the incidence of this disease, but patients are still occasionally seen due to the lack of proper immunization.

❍ **Discuss the differential diagnosis of a patient with muscular dystrophy.**

The differential diagnosis of a specific type of muscular dystrophy is usually based on clinical findings. MYOTONIC DYSTROPHY is the only myopathy characterized by distal muscle weakness. Findings other than myotonia include temporalis and masseter atrophy which causes a skull-like facies, cataracts, testicular atrophy and premature frontal baldness in males. Common to all muscular dystrophies is sparing of the neck extensors, gastrocnemius, posterior tibial and toe flexors. DUCHENNE'S MUSCULAR DYSTROPHY is characterized by early unique involvement of the anterior neck flexors, sternocleidomastoid, anterior abdominal muscles, gluteus medius and tensor fasciae latae. In the shoulder, the lower and middle trapezius are involved, as are the rhomboids, lattissimus dorsi and internal rotators. The hamstrings in Duchenne's are uniquely spared, which is an important finding. In LIMB-GIRDLE MUSCULAR DYSTROPHY, the early unique involvement is mainly the iliopsoas. Other muscles that tend to be involved early are the lower and middle trapezius, rhomboids, latissimus dorsi and internal rotators of the shoulder. The gluteus maximus and the hip abductors are involved in the lower extremities. Uniquely, the brachioradialis is spared early in limb-girdle dystrophy. FASCIOSCAPULOHUMERAL DYSTROPHY is characterized by unique early involvement of the upper pectoralis major and anterior tibialis muscles. There is more sparing early on in this disease than in any other type of dystrophy.

❍ **Discuss the diagnosis of a patient with Guillain-Barré syndrome.**

Guillain-Barré is a neuromuscular disease of acute onset and short duration characterized by acute demyelination of the anterior ramus or motor division of the spinal cord. The posterior ramus and the sensory division of the anterior horn are involved by retrograde extension only. Clinically, patients present with flaccid paralysis which usually begins in the upper extremities. Bulbar involvement may cause respiratory paralysis necessitating tracheostomy. Characteristically the patient is bedfast for 5 to 8 weeks and 3 to 12 months elapsing before they are able to regain enough function to be independent. Recovery continues over the next year and is considered to have plateaued when the motor development does not change over a 16 month period of time. In children the prognosis is worse. Weak dorsiflexors with equines deformity is one of the more characteristic problems. If there is no return in 4 months there probably will be no return. Poor intrinsic hand function is the most frequent upper extremity residual.

❍ **Patients with dermatomyositis have an increased risk of:**

Cancer especially of the lung, gynecologic, prostate, and gastrointestinal which ranges from 5% to 50% in dermatomyositis.

❍ **Describe the management of inflammatory myopathies.**

The management involves pharmacologic agents such as prednisone and immunosuppressants and physical therapy.

❍ **Name some of the causes of diseases occurring at the neuromuscular junction.**

Myasthenia gravis, post polio syndrome, botulinum toxin, nerve gas, and insecticide all affect the neuromuscular junction directly.

○   **How does myasthenia gravis affect the neuromuscular junction?**

Both presynaptically and postsynaptically.

○   **How is the diagnosis of myasthenia gravis made?**

Diagnosis of myasthenia gravis is based on a positive Tensilon test and the presence of serum antibodies.

○   **What is the pharmacologic treatment of myasthenia gravis?**

Pharmacologic treatment for myasthenia gravis includes anticholinesterase inhibitors and immunosuppressants.

○   **What is the cause of post polio syndrome?**

Post polio syndrome is caused by inadequate transmission at the neuromuscular junction.

○   **What are the major categories of peripheral nerve diseases?**

Focal, systemic, demyelinating or axonal.

○   **In partial sciatic nerve injuries, which of the two divisions of the sciatic nerve is most affected?**

The two divisions of the sciatic nerve are the peroneal nerve and the tibial nerve. In partial sciatic nerve injuries the peroneal nerve is usually more severely affected, thus foot drop is almost always more common than calcaneal gait in peripheral nerve injuries.

○   **Why is the peroneal nerve usually more severely affected than the tibial nerve in partial injuries of the sciatic nerve?**

The peroneal nerve is more peripheral than the tibial nerve making it more vulnerable to injuries by injection. The peroneal nerve is has less fibrous tissue protecting it. The peroneal nerve is injured more easily than the tibial nerve and even when both nerves are injured, the peroneal nerve is slower to heal.

○   **What type of nerve disease is Guillain-Barré syndrome?**

Inflammatory neuropathy, systemic with demyelinating and axonal components.

○   **What are the clinical manifestations of Guillain-Barré syndrome?**

Usually acute onset with weakness, atrophy, and sensory loss.

○   **What is the most common peripheral neuropathy?**

Diabetic peripheral neuropathy.

○   **Describe diabetic peripheral neuropathy.**

Diabetic peripheral neuropathy involves all extremities, with the distal lower extremities being involved first. It is a stocking glove distribution with the sensory component more severe than the motor component. It is an axonal neuropathy.

O **What is the isolated severe involvement of only a few nerves with relative sparing of other nerves which occurs in diabetes mellitus known as?**

Mononeuropathy multiplex.

O **What are some diseases associated with immune peripheral neuropathies?**

Rheumatoid arthritis, systemic lupus erythematosus, polyarteritis nodosa, amyloidosis.

O **How is the diagnosis of immune peripheral neuropathy made?**

Diagnosis is based upon clinical presentation, electrodiagnosis, and frequently requires biopsy of nerve and muscle especially for chronic forms.

O **What is the treatment for immune peripheral neuropathy?**

Treatment is pharmacological and depends upon specific etiology, but typically includes nonsteroidal anti-inflammatory drugs, prednisone, and other mmunosuppressants. Plasma exchange may benefit some patients.

O **What is the most common inherited peripheral neuropathy?**

Charcot Marie Tooth Disease also known as hereditary motor sensory neuropathy (HMSN).

O **Describe Hereditary Motor Sensory Neuropathy (HMSN) Type I.**

HMSN I is a hypertrophic and demyelinating neuropathy which results in significantly slowed nerve conduction velocity. Inheritance is autosomal dominant.

O **Describe Hereditary Motor Sensory Neuropathy (HMSN) Type II.**

HMSN II is a predominately axonal neuropathy with only minimal slowing of nerve conduction velocities, but with significant reduction of evoked potential amplitudes. Inheritance is autosomal dominant.

O **Describe Hereditary Motor Sensory Neuropathy (HMSN) Type III.**

HMSN Type III also known as Dejerine-Sottas Disease is a severe demyelinating nonprogressive neuropathic disease that manifests itself in infancy. Weakness is diffuse and more pronounced distally. Motor milestones are delayed. Inheritance is dominant and recessive.

O **Name the Hereditary sensory neuropathies.**

Friedreich's ataxia, ataxia telangiectasia, Tangier's disease and Fabry's disease. These diseases are rare hereditary diseases and characterized by ataxia, long tract signs, cardiovascular disease, and visceral involvement.

O **Where is the level of Cauda Equina Syndrome?**

Intraspinal peripheral nerves at or below L1. The spinal cord ends at the L1 level and injuries at or below L1 affect the cauda equina nerves. Since the nerves are not actually part of the spinal cord, lesions of the cauda equina regenerate and heal as peripheral nerve injury. Thus a person with cauda equina syndrome may have total paralysis from the waist down, but with time and physical therapy, the nerves will regenerate and the person will walk again. This is in contrast with lesions of the spinal cord itself which are part of the central nervous system and do not regenerate.

❍ **What are the clinical patterns of spinal cord disease?**

Depending on the level and type of injury, they may be upper motor neuron, lower motor neuron, or mixed.

❍ **Describe the Spinal Muscle Atrophies.**

Spinal Muscular Atrophy (SMA) type I (known as Werdnig-Hoffman) and SMA type II, affect the anterior horn cell of the spinal cord directly. They manifest themselves in infancy and in early childhood and result in early death. SMA type III (Kugelberg-Welander) occurs much later in childhood and progresses more slowly. SMA type IV is the adult onset Spinal Muscular Atrophy with onset in the third to fifth decades. The disease is slowly progressive and life span is unaffected.

❍ **How are the Spinal Muscular Atrophies diagnosed?**

Diagnosis is based on clinical presentation and confirmed by neuropathic electromyography and biopsy.

❍ **Describe amyotrophic lateral sclerosis (ALS).**

ALS (Lou Gehrig's disease) is an adult motor neuron disease which is a nonfamilial disease of middle age. Distal extremity weakness, particularly in the hands, is a frequent presenting complaint. Weakness progresses proximally and patients eventually have cranial (bulbar) involvement. Muscle fasciculations and atrophy are common. Upper motor neuron findings include hyperreflexia.

❍ **How is Amyotrophic Lateral Sclerosis diagnosed?**

Diagnosis is based on clinical presentation and electrodiagnosis and biopsy confirms a neuropathic process.

❍ **What is the course of Amyotrophic Lateral Sclerosis?**

The disease is progressive and death occurs 3 to 5 years after diagnosis.

❍ **What are the sequelae of postoperative meningomyelocele?**

Leg-length discrepancies, contractures, severe atrophy, sensory deficits, neurogenic bowel and bladder.

❍ **How does intracranial disease affect the lower extremity?**

Generally with spasticity. Middle cerebral artery lesions affect the distal extremity muscles. Anterior cerebral artery lesions affect the proximal extremity muscles.

❍ **What is the most common cause of intracranial disease in children?**

Cerebral palsy.

❍ **What type of cerebral palsy is seen in premature babies?**

Spastic diplegia.

❍ **What is the cause of spastic diplegia cerebral palsy?**

Paraventricular ischemia/hemorrhage.

❍ **Name some examples of acquired intracranial pathology.**

Stroke, brain injury, multiple sclerosis, brain tumor.

O   **What is the distribution of muscle weakness in neuropathy?**

Distal weakness.

O   **What are the electrodiagnostic findings in myopathic diseases?**

Small polyphasic potentials with a myopathic (early) recruitment pattern and if severe, positive waves and fibrillation potentials.

O   **What does the Nerve Conduction Velocity (NCV) Study consist of?**

The NCV consists of the generation of the sensory nerve action potential (SNAP) of sensory nerves and the compound muscle action potential (CMAP) of motor nerves. This study consists of the application of a burst of electrical current to the skin or soft tissue overlying a peripheral nerve and recording of the subsequent compound action potential from the skin or soft tissue overlying the nerve at a distant site.

O   **What is the cause of arthrogryposis?**

Early intrauterine paralysis.

O   **What is spasticity?**

"Spasticity" means that stretch reflexes limit the range and speed of movement due to an upper motor neuron lesion. Because the muscles are never able to lengthen fully they grow less than they should and fixed deformity develops. The bones become abnormally shaped.

O   **What is the incidence of cerebral palsy?**

About 2 per thousand live births.

O   **What are the basic kinds of cerebral palsy?**

Spastic diplegia is paralysis of both legs and is the most common pattern for premature and low birth weight infants. Spastic diplegic occurs shortly after birth. Total body involvement affects speech, trunk, feeding and arms with no walking potential.

O   **Describe the "Total body involvement" pattern of cerebral palsy.**

The cause is due to birth asphyxia or prenatal encephalopathy. These children never walk and have difficulty swallowing and feeding is difficult and slow. They are thin. Gastric reflux may cause choking and aspiration pneumonia. They may require diapering. They have no balance and cannot sit up independently. The limbs remain immobile and contractures develop rapidly. The incidence of hip dislocation and scoliosis is greater than 50%.

O   **What happens in spina bifida?**

In spina bifida the neural tube fails to close during the 4th week. There is paralysis of the legs, anesthesia, and bowel and bladder paralysis to some degree. If the cord supplying the legs is destroyed there is complete flaccid paralysis.

O   **What is the incidence of spina bifida?**

1 in 700 babies are born with spina bifida. The chance of having a second baby with spina bifida is 1 in 40.

O   **What tests prenatally can detect spina bifida?**

Alpha-fetoprotein determination in maternal blood and amniotic fluid, and ultrasound.

O   **How is the neurological deficit classified in spina bifida?**

Spina bifida is classified by the level of the lesion. The level of the last functioning root is used to describe the level of the paraplegia. For example, if L1 is the last working root, the child is described as having L1 paraplegia.

O   **Why is there an overlap between the central nervous system and the peripheral nervous system?**

There is overlap because the spinal cord is classically part of the central nervous system, but contains elements of the peripheral nervous system (e.g., the anterior horn cells or nerve roots).

O   **A painful sensation of tingling, burning, or cold is known as:**

Dysesthesia.

O   **What is a painful sensation caused by non-noxious stimuli, for example, bed sheets rubbing against the feet producing severe pain in patients with peripheral neuropathy.**

Allodynia.

O   **What is the Medical Research Council (MRC) scale of muscle strength that was developed during World War II?**

This is a system for grading muscle strength which is used quite universally although there have been criticisms and the system does not work well with spastic individuals. It is described below:
    5 = full muscle power
    4 = resistance against force
    3 = resistance against gravity but not force
    2 = movement with gravity eliminated
    1 = Flicker of movement or twitch
    0 = no movement

O   **What is paraparesis, back pain, and urinary retention most frequently associated with?**

Spinal cord disease.

O   **What is bilateral foot pain, numbness, and weakness in a distribution of a peripheral nerve associated with?**

Peripheral neuropathy.

O   **What are some causes of disuse atrophy?**

Both nervous pathology and non nervous pathology can result in disuse atrophy. Immobility by casting, bedrest, arthritis, and stroke can all result in disuse atrophy.

O   **What is clonus?**

Clonus is the repetitive movement of a hand, foot, or similar body part when the tendon is stretched. It is an UMN sign. Sometimes patients complain that: "My foot shakes when I walk."

O   **What is the Babinski sign?**

The Babinski sign indicates disease of the UMN system. It is characterized by the rise of the great toe when the lateral plantar aspect of the foot is scratched.

O   **Ipsilateral absent ankle jerk, gastrocnemius atrophy and weakness mostly in plantarflexion suggests?**

S1 nerve root lesion.

O   **What are the hallmark features of peripheral neuropathy?**

Numbness, tingling, pain, weakness, and areflexia. Atrophy occurs when the condition is severe or prolonged.

O   **What causes a demyelinating neuropathy?**

A demyelinating neuropathy is caused by loss or destruction of myelin. The weakness and sensory loss may be proximal or distal, depending on the site of demyelination.

O   **What is the most common cause of acute demyelination?**

Guillain-Barré Syndrome.

O   **What is a widespread neuropathy in which only a few peripheral nerves are affected?**

Mononeuropathy multiplex.

O   **What is a classic pathologic process associated with mononeuropathy multiplex?**

Vasculitis.

O   **What are the characteristic features of radiculopathies?**

In radiculopathies, the pain is usually positional, worse while standing or with prolonged sitting, and improved in the supine position. Increasing the intra-abdominal pressure by coughing, sneezing, or the Valsalva maneuver aggravates the pain. Sensory loss is in a dermatomal distribution and weakness is in a myotomal distribution. Radiculopathies generally cause more pain than weakness and occur in young adults.

O   **What are characteristics of anterior horn cell disorders?**

They cause painless weakness.

O   **What is the most common anterior horn cell disease in adults?**

Amyotrophic lateral sclerosis.

O   **What are the basic characteristics of spinal cord diseases?**

Myelopathies or diseases of the spinal cord, typically cause limb weakness, sensory symptoms, urinary incontinence, and back pain. Pure spinal cord disease is usually spastic.

O   **What is Reflex Sympathetic Dystrophy?**

Reflex sympathetic dystrophy is defined as continuous pain in a portion of an extremity after trauma that may include fracture but does not involve a major nerve associated with sympathetic hyperactivity.

○   **What are some signs of Reflex Sympathetic Dystrophy?**

Atrophy of skin on arms and leg, cool, red, and clammy skin, disuse atrophy of deep structures.

ONYCHCOLOGY

○ **Name the slightly thickened skin just below the free edge of the nail plate. It represents the accumulated keritinocytes streaming distally from the superficial surface of the nail bed.**

Hyponychium.

○ **What is abnormal separation or loosening of the nail plate from the nail bed called?**

Onycholysis.

○ **What the name of the scarring nail dystrophy characteristic of lichen planus?**

Pterygium formation.

○ **Who first described clubbing of the fingernails as an associated clinical sign of thoracic empyema?**

Hippocrates.

○ **What is the most common cause of onychoschizia?**

Repetitive cycles of wetting and drying of the nail plate is the most common cause of onychoschizia or superficial distal lamellar nail splitting.

○ **Which dermatophyte is chiefly responsible for white superficial onychomycosis?**

Trichophyton mentagrophytes.

○ **How is the clinical severity of nail clubbing measured?**

Lovibond's lateral profile sign is used to measure clubbing and is defined as the angle between the curved nail plate and the proximal nail fold. This angle is normally 160 degrees but exceeds 180 degrees in clubbing.

○ **In which racial group is longitudinal melanonychia rarely found?**

Caucasians.

○ **Periungual fibromas or Koenen's tumors are found in 50% of the cases of which disease?**

Tuberous sclerosis.

○ **Myxoid cysts or synovial cysts of the distal dorsal fingers are associated with which type of arthritis?**

Osteoarthritis.

○ **Which diagnostic test is considered the "gold standard" for detecting a glomus tumor of the nail bed?**

Arteriography.

O **What diagnosis should be considered if a streak of longitudinal melanonychia widens?**

Subungual melanoma.

O **How fast should a partial subungual hematoma grow out or move distally?**

At a rate of one millimeter per month.

O **Relative to nail unit pathology, what is Hutchinson's sign?**

A brown to black discoloration of the nail bed "leaking" or spreading to the surrounding nail fold skin sternly suggesting melanoma.

O **What is the medical term for "spoon shaped" nails?**

Koilonychia.

O **What is the medical term for nail biting?**

Onychophagia.

O **What is the medical term for increased curvature of the nail plate along the long axis of the nail unit?**

Platonychia.

O **What is the medical term for fusing of the distal nail plate to the underlying hyponychium and the nail bed?**

Pterygium inversus unguium.

O **What is the medical term for rough nails?**

Trachyonychia.

O **What is the medical term for complete shedding of the nail plate?**

Onychomadesis.

O **What is the medical term for calloused nail groove or nail lip?**

Onychophosis.

O **What is the medical term for spontaneous longitudinal splitting or breaking of the nail plate?**

Onychorrhexis.

O **What is the medical term for neurotic picking at the nails?**

Onychotillomania.

O **What poisoning can cause transverse white bands in the nail plate?**

Arsenic (Mee's lines).

❍   **What is the most common cause of isolated splinter hemorrhages of the nail bed?**

Trauma.

❍   **Which specific form of onychomycosis is associated with infection by the human immunodeficiency virus?**

Proximal subungual onychomycosis.

❍   **In onychomycosis, how long should one wait to see the full therapeutic effect of a three month course of oral itraconazole or terbinafine?**

Ten months.

❍   **Chronic paronychia in a diabetic is most likely caused by which organism?**

Candida.

❍   **Which organism is responsible for over 90% of the cases of onychomycosis?**

Trichophyton rubrum.

❍   **Which is the most sensitive laboratory test for onychomycosis?**

Nail clip biopsy with PAS (periodic acid Schiff) stain.

❍   **What are shallow transverse grooves of the nail plate called?**

Beau's lines.

PHYSICAL MEDICINE AND REHABILITATION

MODALITIES

○ **What is cryotherapy?**

The therapeutic use of cold in the treatment and rehabilitation of musculoskeletal injuries and conditions.

○ **What are the general therapeutic effects of cold therapy?**

Vasoconstriction (reduce bleeding, etc.)
Vasodilatation (rebound dilatation which brings in nutrients, eliminates wastes from the injured area).
Reduce or slow nerve conduction.
Reduce muscle spasm or spasticity.
Reduce tissue metabolism.
Reduce pain.

○ **What is the "Hunting Reaction?"**

Rebound vasodilatation following cold application to preserve tissue viability and prevent tissues from falling below a critical temperature. This is a rewarming phenomenon or reactive hyperemia. It should be noted that early in the post-injury period where there is a tendency to bleed due to vascular disruption, following cold therapy, the area should always be elevated and compressed with some form of compressive device (ie. elastic bandage, Jones compression, etc.) to prevent post-cryotherapy swelling due to the rebound vasodilatation.

○ **What are the subjective phases of ice therapy?**

First is coldness.
Second is burning/pain.
Third is aching/pain.
Fourth is numbness.

○ **How does cold application reduce muscle spasm/spasticity?**

By a direct activity on the muscle spindle producing reduced muscle spindle excitability.

○ **What is the Hoffman or H Response?**

An initial but temporary increase in reflex muscle tone following cold application, possibly secondary to increased alpha motor neuron activity through stimulation of skin sensory receptors. This is, however, temporary and there is an ultimate decrease in muscle tone from cooling of the tissues.

○ **How does tissue cooling reduce pain?**

There may be a number of mechanisms:
- direct effect on sensory nerve endings and pain carrying fibers
- secondary to reduction of muscle spasm
- secondary to limiting bleeding and edema with lower tissue pressures

- secondary to limiting the inflammatory response
- ? influence on the spinal gating mechanism
- ? enhancing endorphin production

○ Which has deeper tissue penetration, superficially applied cold or superficially applied heat?

Superficially applied cold has a significantly greater penetrating power than superficially applied heat. Fat seems to be a better insulator against heating from the outside and once, penetrated through the fat layer, cold seems to be maintained in deeper structures longer than heat. Tissues tend to cool themselves following heat application better than heating themselves after cold application. Vasodilatation more rapidly cools warm tissue than warms cool tissue.

○ What would be some contraindications to the use of cold therapy?

Local ischemic conditions; Raynaud's; Cold allergy; Impaired sensory perception; Possibly - post polio, hypertension.

○ What are different methods of cryotherapy application?

Ice packs/compresses/ice bag
Ice bath.
Ice massage (ice cups, ice cubes, "Popsicles").
Cold sprays (limited effectiveness for typical cryotherapy uses).

○ How long should cold be applied to be effective?

Generally at least 10 minutes of application is needed to be able to reach muscular levels. However, this depends on the status and thickness of the intervening tissues. A good indicator is to generally cool the area to the point of numbness, passing through all 4 subjective cold phases which may take a shorter or longer time depending on the method of cryotherapy used.

○ How long should one utilize cryotherapy before initiating heat therapy?

Heat should never be used in situations which may produce more bleeding/hemorrhage such as for the first couple days following an injury. On the other hand, because of the deep penetrating power of cold and the resulting vasodilatation which occurs following cold therapy, some practitioners may not go to typical heat applications at all and get the same healing benefits of deep vasodilatation from application of cold.

○ What are "contrast baths?"

This is a combined, alternating use of cold and heat during the same treatment session. Depending on the protocol, you may start with cold and end with cold or in some instances, start with cold and end with heat. The times may be 1-2 minutes cold and perhaps 4-6 minutes heat. When completing one phase, ie., cold, the extremity is immediately submerged in the heat for the appropriate time. When done with the heat, the extremity is immediately submerged in the cold. This is done with alternating cold and heat for 30-45 minutes. This tends to produce a constriction-dilatation-constriction-dilatation activity which may produce a "milking" action on post-traumatic edema and would, therefore, be appropriate to use in situations involving swelling due to trauma. Care should be taken to avoid using heat in situations where vasodilatation would increase the swelling, ie., in the immediate post-injury period of a couple days.

○ What are the different forms of heat or thermotherapy?

Conductive heat.
Convective heat.

Conversive heat.

O   **What is an example of "conductive" heat?**

The typical example of conductive heat may be hot packs or paraffin therapy. In conductive heat, the heat from an object which is placed ON the skin is "conducted" from the source to the cooler body.

O   **What is an example of "convective" heat?**

An example of convective heat is whirlpool, fluidotherapy and ultraviolet therapy. In convective heat, the heat source is "projected" toward the skin surface and basically creates a swirling or convection around the object being treated.

O   **What is an example of "conversive" heat?**

Specific examples of conversive heat would be ultrasound, diathermy or infrared therapy in which the heating effect is produced by a conversion of one energy form to heat as it passes through the tissues.

O   **What are some of the physiologic effects of heat/thermotherapy?**

Physiologic effects of heat/thermotherapy are:
- vasodilatation (active hyperemia) with increased blood flow increased capillary
  permeability with increased exchange of materials between tissue and
  circulation (nutrients/wastes and byproducts)
- increased exchange of oxygen and carbon dioxide between tissues and blood
- increased metabolism (healing effect with production of proteins, etc.)
- increased collagen extensibility to improve ROM and decrease stiffness and
  adhesions
- muscle relaxation by reduction of muscle spindle excitability
- sedation
- analgesia

O   **What is the advantage of conversive heat over conductive and convective heat?**

Conversive heat has the potential of greater/deeper tissue penetration as it penetrates and becomes converted to heat. Both conductive and convective forms of heat have very minimal tissue penetration, generally less than 4-5 mm with the fat layer being a relatively effective barrier against penetration. Therefore, to obtain deep heating effects, conversive heat methods must be applied.

O   **What would be some contraindications to the use of heat/thermotherapy?**

Acute trauma.
Advanced PVD (steal phenomenon).
Patients with heat sensitivity.
Patients with heat insensitivity.
Febrile conditions.
        -Conditions where vasodilatation may exacerbate exudation of fluids or interfere with blood flow.
        - Over malignancies or in extremes in age.

O   **How should "hot packs" be applied?**

The hot pack which is a gel filled cloth pack is heated to 140-170 degrees in a hydrocolator. The hot pack should NOT be placed directly on the skin but wrapped in about 8 layers of terry cloth and then applied to the surface. The treatment time is usually about 20-30 minutes at which time the hot pack has lost sufficient temperature by conduction to the body to be of no further effect. The hot pack supplies "moist" heat.

○   How is a paraffin bath administered?

A paraffin and mineral oil mixture is heated to 122-138 degrees and the extremity is "dipped" 6-13 times into the paraffin bath and removed, allowing each successive layer to harden. When the extremity has been dipped a sufficient number of times, the extremity is wrapped in plastic or waxed paper and covered with a towel and maintained in this wrap for 20-30 minutes after which the wrap and paraffin may be removed. Paraffin may be particularly good for arthritic conditions, tendonitis and bursitis and should not be used in situations involving open wounds or ulcers, active dermatitis, PVD or in patients with decreased sensation.

○   How is hydrotherapy applied?

Hydrotherapy (whirlpool) is a form of convective heat. In warm whirlpool the temperature of the water should be between 98-102 degrees and the warm heat in conjunction with the water agitation provides a mild heating and massaging effect. The temperature should be lower in the elderly, the very young patient, and patients with PVD or with sensation abnormalities, i.e. Diabetes Mellitus. The treatment time is generally 20-30 minutes.

○   What is "ultrasound" and how is the heat produced?

Ultrasound is a form of conversive heat. The ultrasound head contains a piezoelectric crystal that emits a sound wave when an electrical current is passed through. This sound wave is of a frequency (.8-1.2 MHz) to pass through tissues. When the sound wave contacts a tissue interface with a difference in density, some of the wave passes through, some is reflected and some converted into heat. Therefore, ultrasound appears to heat best at areas of greater variance in tissue density, ie. going from a lower density to a higher density (muscle/fat to tendon/ligament/capsule) or going from a higher density to a lower density. However the denser the tissue, the more resistance so ultrasound is best used around tissue of high density (ligament, capsule, tendon, fibrotic/scarred areas).

○   What are the general tissue effects of ultrasound?

Heating effect – the absorption of the energy by tissue resistance produces heat. The greater the energy absorbed, the greater the heating effect which is a function of both the frequency and the intensity of the wave.

Mechanical effect – the sound "vibrations" produce a cavitation effect producing slits between intermolecular bonds resulting in the breakdown of scar and adhesion and decreased joint fluid viscosity.

Chemical/cellular effects – effects include increase enzyme activity, increased cell membrane permeability, increased local blood flow, decreased metabolite build up and decreased muscular spasm.

○   How is ultrasound applied?

The ultrasound can be applied by direct contact to the skin using a "coupling medium" such as mineral oil or a commercial gel which promotes a good coupling of the ultrasound head to the skin to maximize the delivery of the wave and to prevent sound wave scatter. The head is moved continuously but slowly (approximately 1 cm/second) to prevent accumulation of heat at any one point. The ultrasound can also be applied underwater, with the water serving as the coupling agent. Underwater the ultrasound head is held about 1 inch away from the skin surface and moved as above. Underwater technique is best used for areas with irregular surface contour to provide an even ultrasound wave. Treatment time in both is about 6-12 minutes. For most Podiatric usage, the intensity of the wave is between 1-1.7 watts/cm2 depending on the thickness of the tissue to be penetrated (the deeper the penetration needed the higher the intensity).

○   Where should ultrasound NOT be used?

Over the spinal cord.
over open epiphyseal plates.
In hemorrhagic conditions or disorders.
Over malignancies or tumors.
Over pacemakers.
Over a pregnant uterus or reproductive organs.
In vascular insufficiency.
Over anesthetic areas.
A relative contraindication would be over metallic implants.

❍   What is diathermy and how does it produce a heating effect?

Diathermy is a form of conversive heating where a form electrical energy is converted into heat energy. In short wave diathermy, a high frequency electrical current produces heat as it passes through tissues by resistance of the current. In microwave diathermy, high frequency electromagnetic radiation produces molecular stimulation as it passes through tissues producing a heating effect.

❍   Which tissues are more greatly affected by diathermy?

Tissues with higher water content such as muscle appear to have the greatest effect of higher tissue temperatures produced with diathermy. However, in fluids with increased polarity, such as synovial fluid and cerebrospinal fluid, the heating is exaggerated with a greater and detrimental temperature elevation and, therefore, diathermy should be avoided over areas with synovial fluid or cerebrospinal fluid.

❍   Which appears to have the greatest heating effect, shortwave or microwave diathermy?

While the effects are similar with similar indications and contraindications, the increase in temperature difference between subcutaneous tissues and muscle appears to be greater in microwave diathermy. Also microwave diathermy continues its heating effect for a number of minutes (up to 20 min) after discontinuing treatment due to the produced molecular stimulation.

❍   What would be some contraindications for the use of diathermy?

Over a pacemaker.
In acute hemorrhagic conditions or with acute trauma.
In patients with heat insensitivity.
Over a pregnant uterus or with menstruation.
Over a area of malignancy.
Over metallic implants.
Over areas of local or systemic infection.
Over open epiphyseal plates.
In patients with PVD.

❍   In forms of conversive heat, what effects should the patient notice?

There should actually be minimal to no heat sensation appreciated in either ultrasound or diathermy and treatments should not produce pain or discomfort.

❍   What is the difference between ultraviolet and infrared light therapy?

Ultraviolet light therapy is a form of radiant heat, ie. sun rays, which when applied to the surface of the skin produces a photochemical effect and erythema producing "sunburn" effect. The radiant heat penetrates to the basal skin layer and is absorbed producing its effects. Infrared light therapy is a form of conversive heat therapy where infrared light, which is invisible, is converted to heat by interaction with tissue. In infrared, the light wave is emitted as photons and the photons are absorbed by the skin and tissues and converted to heat.

○   **What is the effect of infrared therapy?**

Infrared therapy provides superficial heating and vasodilatation. The effect is only a couple mm in depth of penetration with heat absorbed in subcutaneous layers and dissipated. IR therapy stimulates cutaneous nerve endings, stimulates superficial capillary circulation and stimulates eccrine sweat glands. There is minimal heat sensation and mild erythema which rapidly clears following discontinuation of the IR source.

○   **What is the effect of ultraviolet radiation therapy?**

The radiant energy produces a lasting erythema or "sunburn" effect with some individuals more sensitive to the ultraviolet radiation (ie. redheads/blonds). The dose is a function of the "MED" or Minimal Erythema Dose or the minimal amount of UV radiation that produces an erythematous reaction. Adverse long term effects of ultraviolet radiation are well known such as the increased incidence of skin malignancies. UV therapy is most used in the treatment of dermatological conditions (granulation tissue, ulcerations, acne, psoriasis) due to its bacteriocidal, fungistatic and vitamin D producing effects.

○   **What are some of the physical benefits to electrical stimulation?**

Pain relief.
Reduction of edema.
Muscle strengthening and re-education.
Osteogenesis.

○   **How does electrical stimulation reduce pain?**

The answer may still be unclear but a number of mechanisms have been proposed:
- Effect on the spinal "Gating" mechanism
- Stimulation of the production of endorphins and enkephalins
- Altered nocireceptor polarity
- Enzymatic degradation of pain substances
- Stimulation of microcirculation.

○   **What are some physiologic effects of cutaneous electrical stimulation?**

Increased circulation with active hyperemia.
Acceleration of lymphatic flow.
Stimulation of cellular function.
Increased ATP production.

○   **What is the difference between high voltage and low voltage electrical stimulator devices?**

High voltage devices use a set high voltage current to overcome areas of variable tissue resistance (impedance). Where there is high resistance, due to "Ohm's Law" there would be lower current and areas of low resistance there would be higher current. Therefore, because a fixed high current is used to overcome areas of high resistance, when areas of low resistance are encountered, the higher current may produce discomfort and may be detrimental to healing. In newer, low voltage devices, a current meter detects impedance (tissue resistance) and the voltage is adjusted according to impedance providing a constant low amp current in a comfortable range and without as detrimental effect to healing.

○   **What is M.E.N.S. therapy?**

M.E.N.S. stands for Microamp Electrical Nerve Stimulation. This form of therapy provides a current in the microamp range. It is believed that microamp currents may have some significant physiological effects such as:

- increasing local ATP production
- restoring membrane transport systems
- stimulating and increasing the inflow of nutrients
- stimulating and increasing the outflow of wastes
- enhancing proteins synthesis
- increase amino acid transport.

M.E.N.S. therapy is comfortable and safe because it is close to physiologic current and produces only rare adverse reactions.

O   How do different electrical frequencies have different effects?

Different frequencies of the electrical current effect different forms of nerve in different ways. Sympathetic nerve is most affected by lower frequency electrical currents in the range of 0-5 Hz and, therefore, produce effects such as edema control with currents of lower frequency. Smooth muscle is best stimulated at currents of 0-10 Hz and, therefore, stimulation at this frequency range may also assist in edema control.

Motor nerve appears to be most effected by currents of 10-50 Hz and, therefore, current in this frequency range would have the greatest effect on muscle stimulation.

Sensory nerve appears to be most effected by currents in the 90 (80) to 110 (150) Hz range and, therefore, current in this frequency may be best used to reduce pain. Nocireceptors appear to be best affected with currents of about 130 Hz as well.

Low frequency waves stimulate smooth muscle (edema control). Intermediate frequency waves stimulate muscle (motor nerve). High frequency waves stimulate sensory nerve producing pain relief.

O   What is the difference between premodulated and interferential electrical stimulation?

In premodulated (bipolar) electrical stimulation, the electrical current consists of a "pre-mixed" set of sine waves with the resultant current a composite of the 2 mixed frequencies, set by the stimulator. 2 electrodes are used and the current flows between the 2 electrodes and treats the intervening area. In interferential (quadripolar) electrical stimulation, 2 pairs of electrodes, each with their own frequency (generally one fixed frequency current and one adjustable frequency current) are arranged so that the 2 currents cross and "interfere" with each other. The 2 mixed currents result in composite current frequency producing a beating effect, deeper stimulation and occurring over a larger area encompassed by the rectangle produced by the 4 electrodes at the 4 corners.

O   What is "Russian Stimulation?"

This is a fixed sinusoidal current of very high frequency (2500 Hz) which produces strong tetanic contractions and used for muscle strengthening and re-education. The stimulation can be adjusted by altering contraction and relaxation cycles of the muscle by changing the frequency of occurrence duration and method in which the current is applied.

O   What may be some contraindications to electrical stimulation?

It should not be used over electronic demand pacemakers or over electrical implants. It should also not be used in cancer patients as well as in areas of thrombophlebitis, epilepsy and cardiac conduction problems. It should not be applied over a pregnant uterus, over the larynx or pharynx, carotid sinus, transthoracically or transcerebrally.

O   What are the mechanical effects of massage therapy?

Production of intramuscular motion to stretch or break adhesions, mobilize fluid accumulations and break up or mobilize deposits. There is no effect on strength.

Circulatory effects by compressing low pressure vessels, thereby augmenting venous and lymphatic return as well as stimulating arteriolar blood moving into the vacated capillary beds. Production of cutaneous hyperemia by mast cell stimulation, histamine release, etc., producing vasodilatation.

O   **How does massage relieve pain?**

It may relieve pain by a variety of mechanisms. Stimulation of superficial receptors which may block transmission of other receptors, ie. pain receptors. Produces sedation/relaxation of muscle spasm. Stimulates the reduction of edema, thereby reducing tissue pressure. Breaks up fibrosis and adhesion/scar which may be a contributing factor to pain.

O   **What are the different basic strokes of massage?**

Effleurage or stroking
Petrissage or compression.
Tapotement or percussion.

O   **How is Effleurage accomplished?**

Effleurage can be composed of light, superficial stroking with light pressure, primarily providing superficial receptor stimulation without much circulatory or mechanical effect or can be deep stroking with greater mechanical effect and stimulation of venous and lymphatic return. Stroking should always be in the direction of venous/lymphatic flow, therefore centripetally or towards the heart.

O   **What are the various forms of Petrissage?**

The typical forms of petrissage are:
- kneading
- squeezing
- friction
- rolling
- shaking

All forms have the tendency to mechanically stimulate and affect deeper tissues, to provide for deeper tissue mobilization.

O   **What is cross fiber massage?**

This is a form of friction massage where compression and friction is provided in short strokes perpendicular to the long axis of the fiber/scar/tendon, etc. This breaks up obliquely lying adhesions and scar and assists in "lining up" collagen fibers and scar in a more orderly, physiologically and anatomically advantageous alignment.

O   **What is Anodyne Monochromatic Infrared Therapy?**

The Anodyne Therapy System is an FDA-cleared infrared medical device that increases circulation and decreases pain. It is used primarily to reduce the pain and restore sensation in diabetic neuropathy.

Rehabilitation Principles

O   **When fitting crutches, how long should the crutches be?**

With the patient standing and the crutch tips slightly ahead of the toes and the crutches angled out 6-10¼ from the body, there should be about 2-3 finger breadths distance (1¼–2¼½) from the axillary pads of the crutches to the axilla for a proper fit. The axillary pads should not be compressed into the axilla and weight should not be borne in the axilla. The axillary pads are stabilized against the chest wall with the upper arm.

❍ What is the proper position/location of the handgrip for crutches, canes and walkers?

With the elbow flexed at about 15-20 degrees and the hand on the handgrip, the grip is at the approximate level of the greater trochanter of the femur.

❍ When stair climbing with crutches in a non-weightbearing gait, what is the correct order of crutches and protected and normal limbs?

When going up stairs, the good, weight-bearing limb goes up first followed by the protected limb and crutches. When going down stairs, the crutches and protected limb go down first followed by the good, weight-bearing limb.

❍ When ambulating with a single cane or single crutch, in which side should the cane or crutch be used?

The cane should be used on the side opposite the protected side, therefore on the normal/good side.

❍ In ambulating with crutches with a non-weight bearing limb, how would you best describe the activity of the weight-bearing limb?

The weight bearing limb should continue in a toe off to heel contact stride with the weight bearing limb swinging through the crutches to maintain a tripod type configuration of the weight bearing limb and the 2 crutch tips.

❍ What are different forms of crutch gait?

Swing through non-weight bearing gait.
 -no weight on involved limb, good limb swings through and bears full weight.
Partial weight bearing, "3 point" gait.
 -partial weight bearing limb remains in line with the crutches, with variable weight bearing, good limb
 swings through.
Full weight bearing, "4 point" gait.
 -cadence is right crutch, left leg (full weight), left crutch, right leg (full weight).
Full weight bearing, "2 point" gait.
 -cadence is right crutch and left leg together, left crutch and right leg together.
Double swing through, weight bearing gait.
 -crutches move forward together, both legs swing through together.

❍ List some methods for ankle protection (immobilization).

Adhesive taping/strapping.
Unna boot/Gelocast.
Prefabricated splints (stirrup splint, lace-up, etc.)
Jones Compression.
Posterior plaster splint, stirrup splint.
Fabricated splints (Orthoplast, etc.)
+/- AFO.
Removable walkers (CAM walker, etc.)
Cast immobilization.

❍ Stirrup splints, i.e., Air-Stirrup, Gel splint, etc. limit motion primarily on the _____ plane while permitting motion on the _____ plane.

Frontal, Sagittal.

○   **What are some limitations or problems with ankle taping/strapping?**

Method and skill of application.
Skin associated problems (tape rash, folliculitis, blisters, etc.)
Frequent applications.
Limit concurrent rehabilitation exercises.
Lose significant support/strength after 15-20 minutes of vigorous activity.
More difficult to self apply.
More costly with frequent/repeated applications than cost of splint.
Bathing/cleansing or requirement to keep tape dry.

○   **What are some advantages and disadvantages of removable BK walkers?**

Advantages:
      Removable to allow for rehabilitation, wound care.
      Comfort and adjustability (snugness, ankle joint ROM).
      Sufficient immobilization (in many cases).
      Reusable, cost effective.
      Fewer problems with application (vs. cast immobilization).
      Generally rocker bottom for easier ambulation.
      Fewer pressure related problems, i.e. peroneal palsy from compression of top edge of cast.
      Can accommodate swelling (reapply).

Disadvantages:
      Can be removed in non-compliant patient.
      If not applied correctly, can result in insufficient immobilization.
      Alter limb lengths.

○   **How are muscles graded/scaled according to manual muscle testing?**

0 = No contraction of muscle.
1 = Contraction of muscle, but no motion.
2 = Contraction, with motion through full range but with gravity eliminated.
3 = Contraction with full range of motion against gravity but with no further resistance.
4 = Contraction with full range of motion with resistance but less resistance than expected normal.
5 = Contraction with full range of motion with full, expected resistance applied.

To achieve a particular grade, the muscle should be able to move a joint through a full range of motion. The grade can be assigned a – or a + if resistance is slightly less or more than expected.

○   **What is the difference between testing a muscle at its "advantaged" vs ."disadvantaged" position?**

To test a muscle at its advantaged position means testing is done with the muscle started at its shortest (contracted/strongest) position and the examiner attempts to overcome or "break" the contraction with their manual resistance. This may be used in muscles which are weaker or with smaller normal ranges of motion but, for the most part is not as acceptable as testing a muscle from its disadvantaged position. To test a muscle at its disadvantaged position means testing starting from its longest (stretched) and initially non-contracted (weakest) state and the examiner provides resistance as the patient contracts the muscle to move it through a full range of motion. This is generally more advantageous, particularly in stronger muscles and muscles with larger ranges of motion. This method allows the examiner to identify areas of weakness, allow better quantification of the strength, identify problem areas, allow better qualification of the strength (alterations in contraction quality and quantity).

○   **What are "end feels" and what do they mean?**

End feels are the quality or character of the end point of range of motion (stopping point) and can assist the examiner in determining what may be limiting or restricting the range of motion.

○   **What are the typical forms of "end feels?"**

Hard (Bony) – typifies bone against bone.

Tension – typifies stretching of dense connective tissue. As more pressure is applied, more tension is generated in the connective tissue, more resistance is encountered by the examiner.

Springy – typifies fibrous tissue, cartilage or fluid within a joint, between the adjacent joint surfaces as a limiting factor to ROM.

Soft – typifies limitation of ROM when 2 soft surfaces abut against each other, such as muscle against muscle (gastro-soleus against hamstrings with knee flexion).

○   **What are different ways to describe "muscle imbalance?"**

Right vs. left imbalance.
Agonist vs. antagonist imbalance (strength ratio imbalance).
Strength vs. flexibility imbalance.

○   **In a rehabilitation program, which physical parameter should be initially addressed to improve the success of an exercise/rehab program?**

The first thing which should be addressed is range of motion. This prevents adhesions/fibrosis, may stimulate healing of tissues (better alignment of collagen, etc.) and allow muscle to be able to be worked or strengthened through as near maximal range of motion as possible.

○   **What is the SAID principle of rehabilitation?**

SAID stands for Specific Adaptation to Imposed Demands which means that a rehabilitation program should be patterned after demands and stresses made upon an individual, encountered during their particular type of activity and that for beneficial and rehabilitative effects to occur, those particular body systems must be specifically and sufficiently stressed for beneficial changes to occur. For example, to gain strength in a particular muscle, that muscle has to be specifically and significantly stressed.

○   **What are the 5 main areas of emphasis in an exercise rehabilitation program?**

Range of motion and flexibility.
Muscle strength.
Muscle endurance.
Cardiovascular endurance.
Neuromuscular coordination (balance, agility, speed, proprioception, reaction time, etc.).

○   **What are the three basic types of stretching/flexibility techniques?**

Ballistic stretching which requires a patient to use their body momentum to stretch or force a muscle into stretch. This employs bouncing type motions. THIS TECHNIQUE SHOULD NEVER BE DONE. The muscle tends to become over stretched which stimulates the myotactic reflex, forcing the muscle to contract, thereby tightening the muscle and leading to a greater incidence of injury. As well, forcing a muscle into stretch by explosive motions results in an increase incidence of muscle strain and rupture.

Static stretching or passive stretching where a muscle is slowly, but continually and incrementally stretched and held in the stretched position for a period of time. This can be done either by the patient themselves or by the practitioner. This employs no ballistic or forced activities or motions. The muscle is slowly placed on stretch and slowly stretched further as the muscle responds and relaxes to the stretch.

Contract-relax stretching involves a passive stretch to tightness, followed by an isometric contraction and relaxation cycle with increased passive stretch during the relaxation period. This contract-relax cycle is repeated 3-4 times.

○ What would be the difference in rehabilitation techniques directed toward muscle strength vs. muscle endurance?

In muscle strength, generally high weight with a low number of repetitions is used. In muscle endurance training, lower weight with a higher number of repetitions is used.

○ What is the difference between isometric, isotonic, and isokinetic exercise?

In **isometric** exercise, the muscle is contracted against a fixed resistance, with no joint motion produced, only stimulating muscle contraction. The tension in the muscle is proportional to the effort supplied by the patient, i.e. more effort, more muscular tension.

In **isotonic** exercise, a weight is moved through a range of motion. While the weight technically does not changed, it may be affected by gravity. The isotonic exercise may be concentric (muscle contracting and getting shorter - also called positive work) or eccentric (muscle contracting and getting longer – also called negative work). Also, not all points in a range of motion are of equal strength with some segments weaker and some stronger. In **isokinetic** exercise, a weight is not used but the patient works against a bar which is speed controlled or limited and can be moved only so fast as set by the examiner. As the patient pushes harder against the bar, while it can move only so fast, the bar provides more resistance. Therefore, with a greater effort against the bar, there is more resistance, therefore, more strengthening effect.

○ What is the "sticking point" and to what does it apply?

The "sticking point" can be defined as the weakest segment in a range of motion. In isotonic exercise, to work through a full range of motion, the maximal weight which can be used is only that which can be moved through this weakest or sticking point. Therefore, maximal benefit may be obtained in this weakest segment of motion by maximal resistance received but less than maximal benefit is obtained in the stronger segments since they are less than maximally challenged or resisted.

○ When rehabilitating a patient to include cardiovascular endurance as well as local rehabilitation, how can the heart rate be of assistance in determining the cardiovascular conditioning stress level?

As cardiovascular stress increases, the heart rate increases. A general tip in calculating the appropriate cardiovascular stress is to get the heart rate into a "training range." This training range is estimated at about 70-85% of ones maximal heart rate. The maximal heart rate can be estimated at about 220 minus the patient's age. Therefore for a 40 year old individual, the estimated training heart range would be 70-85% of 220-40 or about 126-153 beats/minute.

○ What is the effect of strength training on proprioceptive training?

For proprioception to be improved, adequate strength is necessary to be able to maintain the correct position of the body and its weight in space. Therefore, strength of fine control muscles must be improved and stressed before specific proprioception exercises can be effectively performed. For example, single limb standing with the eyes open works on improving fine muscular control with the assistance of visual coordination, the vestibular apparatus as well as some proprioceptive input. But to selectively improve proprioception, once this fine muscular control is adequate, single limb standing with the eyes close provides greater stress on the peripheral proprioceptive apparatus due to absence of visual input.

O   **When developing a rehabilitative exercise program for a patient, what are some principles to which the program should adhere?**

Try to work at as full a range of motion as possible.

Muscular exercises should be performed slowly, smoothly and under control without jerking or excessively rapid motions.

The exercise should produce minimal or no pain. Attention should be directed towards stressing particular muscles or muscle groups in need.

The resistance provided should be sufficient but not so excessive that the patient cannot complete an exercise or of a magnitude that cannot safely be controlled by the patient.

Both sides (left and right) and agonists and antagonists should be exercised.

Therapeutic exercises should maintain or restore correct balance between agonist and antagonist muscle groups.

The patient should adhere to a regular and sufficiently frequent schedule.

PODOPEDIATRICS

○ **What specific radiographic finding is seen in lead poisoning in pediatric bone?**

Dense white transverse bands in metaphysis.

○ **What blood test during pregnancy is an indicator of neurological problems for the fetus?**

Elevated Alpha-fetal protein.

○ **What birth presentation may account for a Congenital Dislocated Hip?**

Breech.

○ **What conditions may show absent phalangeal epiphyses?**

Hypothyroidism, Trisomy 18, and Edwards syndrome.

○ **Osteochondrosis of the talus is called?**

Diaz Mouchet.

○ **Os Trigonum is what structure before it is an accessory bone?**

Secondary Ossification center of talus.

○ **What is the name of the classical sign on lateral radiograph of the navicular in Köhler's?**

Dime sign.

○ **What significant eye problem should be assessed in a patient with Pauciarticular Juvenile Arthritis?**

Iridocyclitis.

○ **What is the most common diagnosis for a child under 5 years old who refuses to stand or walk and spontaneously gets better in 3-5days with no treatment?**

Transient Synovitis.

○ **What is the sex and age predilection for Pauci Articular Juvenile Arthritis?**

Girls under 5 years old.

○ **What is the expected normal value for the metatarsus adductus angle on A-P view of a 6 month old infant?**

20-25 degrees adduction.

○ **What is the upper limit for the acetabular index on frog leg lateral view in a neonate?**

25 degrees.

⭘   **What is the name of constrictive bands of tissue around the foot and leg in T.E.V.?**

Streeter's Dysplasia.

⭘   **Constriction of what structure might cause damage to the femoral head during treatment for C.D.H?**

Ligament Capitus Femorus i.e. Nutrient artery of femoral head.

⭘   **What immunization has been linked as a causative agent in Juvenile Septic Arthritis?**

Rubella.

⭘   **When observing a child less than 2 years old with a Toddler fracture the best radiographic view would be?**

Anterior Posterior view of tibia.

⭘   **What specific Biomechanical finding might you expect on lower extremity evaluation of a 10 year old child who had a Pauciarticular Arthritis of the ankle at 3 years of age?**

Limb length discrepancy on affected limb.

⭘   **When evaluating an A-P view of a 6-year-old child with metatarsus adductus where would you observe the position of the navicular?**

Lateral to talar head.

⭘   **What position of the talus to calcaneus would you observe on a lateral radiograph of a patient with Talipes EquinoVarus?**

Talus parallel to calcaneus.

⭘   **If you observed a positive Barlow's Test on an infant, what would be the next hip test you would perform?**

Ortolani's Test.

⭘   **What test would you perform on a 5-year-old child who you suspect of a Congenital Dislocated Hip?**

Galeazzi's Or Allis Test.

⭘   **While evaluating a Frog Lateral Radiograph of 6-month-old child, you note that the femoral heads are above Hilgenreiner's Line. What does this say about baby's hip?**

Normal Hip.

⭘   **What range of motion, during a hip examination in a neonate, would lead you to the diagnosis of a Congenital Dislocated Hip?**

Limited abduction of flexed thigh.

○ **At what phase of gait is a Twister Cable effective?**

Swing phase.

○ **What tests for flat foot best demonstrate if the foot can form an arch?**

Jack's or Hubscher Tests.

○ **What specific surgical procedure might be recommended for a painful calcaneal- navicular coalition?**

Cowell Procedure.

○ **What familial anatomical etiology best explains a structural intoe, which never reduces?**

Acetabular position is internal and anterior.

○ **What is the name of the inherited condition of absence of 2nd, 3rd and 4th toes and metatarsals giving a cleft in the forefoot?**

Ectrodactyly.

○ **What factor of acetabular dysplasia may account for a Congenital Dislocated Hip?**

Anterior displacement on pelvis.

○ **At what time period does a normal baby 1st sit up unassisted?**

6 months postpartum.

○ **What effect does hypothyroidism have on pediatric bone?**

Delayed ossification.

○ **What is the appearance of the epiphysis on a radiograph in the regenerative stage of osteochondrosis?**

Fragmentation of the epiphysis.

○ **According to Rushford what percentage of infants with metatarsus adductus spontaneously corrects?**

86%.

○ **What iatrogenic problem can occur with derotational casting for clubfoot by aggressive dorsiflexion for the equinus component?**

Vertical Talus.

○ **Why is a Pavlik Harness a preferred treatment for an infant with a Congenital Dislocatable Hip?**

Infant can kick and move legs.

○ **How do you determine the proper size of a Denis Browne Bar?**

A.S.I.S. to A.S.I.S. plus 2 inches or Acromion to Acromion.

○ **What is the classical presentation observed in a Talipes Calcaneal Valgus foot in newborn nursery?**

Dorsal foot is dorsiflexed to tibia, heel in valgus off weight bearing, and forefoot abductus.

○ **What is the normal value for internal torsion of the femur in a neonate?**

25-30 degrees internal.

○ **What anatomical factor accounts for the appearance of a tibial varum in children less than 18 months old?**

Lateral position of gastrosoleus muscles to tibia.

○ **Why are gait plates usually discontinued by age 10?**

Sesamoids form and usually cause sesamoiditis with gait plate use.

○ **What chromosome has been identified in Ehlers-Danlos Syndrome?**

Chromosome 15.

○ **What presentation is seen in the hands of a child with Marfan's Syndrome?**

Arachnodactyly.

○ **What symptomatic tarsal coalition has the greatest incidence in the pediatric foot?**

Talo-calcaneal coalition.

○ **What is a characteristic feature of an athetoid cerebral palsy patient?**

Dysarthria.

○ **When is hand preference normal in a child?**

Approximately 24 months of age.

○ **What is a characteristic presentation for the leg in Charcot Marie Tooth Syndrome?**

Stork leg or inverted champagne bottle appearance.

○ **What is the name given to a syndactyly of 2nd and 3rd digits?**

Zygodactyly.

○ **What dwarfism shows a hallux varus (hitchhikers sign) in the newborn nursery?**

Diastrophic dwarfism.

○ **Why was the Harris Beath view first used?**

Evaluate rigid flat feet in Army recruits with medial or posterior calcaneal facet coalitions.

RADIOLOGY, IMAGING, RADIATION PROTECTION AND SAFETY

○ **On radiographic analysis, the bones of one foot demonstrate a flowing "candle-wax" hyperostosis adhering to a sclerotomal pattern of distribution. The most likely diagnosis is:**

Melorheostosis.

○ **The radiographic hallmark of hyperparathyroidism is:**

Subperiosteal resorption.

○ **Of adult rheumatoid arthritis, systemic lupus, seronegative arthritis, and sarcoidosis, in which of these disorders is acrosclerosis unusual?**

Adult rheumatoid arthritis.

○ **Solid periosteal reactions are the radiographic hallmark of:**

Benign processes.

○ **In conventional radiography, the four determinants of subject contrast are:**

Thickness, density, atomic number and kilovoltage.

○ **Increasing the mAs by 15% will have what predicted effect on contrast**

None.

○ **Decreasing the kilovoltage will have what predicted effect on contrast**

Increase contrast.

○ **Increasing the kilovoltage by 15% will have what predicted effect on film density**

Density is approximately doubled.

○ **The presence of medullary sclerosis in known osteomyelitis suggests:**

Chronicity.

○ **On a standard x-ray machine control console, the milliamperage controls the**

Tube current.

○ **Filtration is required by law because it functions by:**

Lowering the skin radiation dose by removing low energy (soft), long wavelength radiation from the x-ray beam.

○   **1 Sievert (Sv) of radiation is equivalent to _____ rems**

100 rems.

○   **The most consistent radiographic feature in the long bones of a pediatric patient with   acute lymphocytic leukemia is?**

Transverse metaphyseal lucent banding.

○   **An adolescent patient presents with ankle pain and swelling and a radiographic pattern of serpiginous pattern of internal osteolysis. This pattern is virtually pathognomic for?**

Acute hematogenous osteomyelitis.

○   **Total fix time generally equals _____ the clearing time:**

Twice or two-times.

○   **Spinal ventosa dactylitis of the hands and feet is the radiographic manifestation of which disorder?**

Tuberculous osteomyelitis in children, although occasionally seen with sickle-cell disease and congenital syphilis.

○   **The 4 basic differentials to be considered in any symptomatic patient with Paget's disease are:**

Osteoarthritis, pathologic fracture or pseudofracture, neurologic impingement, or malignant degeneration.

○   **Osteoid osteomas are most frequently encountered in which foot bone?**

The talus.

○   **Osteochondromas should be distinguished radiographically from bizarre osteochondromatous proliferations. The key distinguishing feature is?**

Osteochondromas demonstrate medullary confluence and metaphyseal flaring with the host bone.

○   **Cystic lesions of the calcaneal body are not uncommonly encountered. The three most frequently encountered biopsy proven lesions are:**

Simple bone cyst, intraosseous lipoma, and aneurysmal bone cyst.

○   **Multiple phleboliths in the presence of a soft tissue mass is strongly suggestive of what pathologic lesion?**

Hemangioma (or other vascular lesion).

○   **Three-phase power x-ray generators produce better images than single-phase power generators because they have what effect on the ripple factor?**

Decrease ripple.

○   **Step-down transformers in conventional x-ray units are necessary in that they?**

Provide low voltage to drive current in the filament circuit (10 volts).

○ **In considering focal spot size, source-image distance (SID), and object-image distance (OID), what must be done to each factor to insure a maximally sharp x-ray image?**

Maximize SID whilst minimizing focal spot size and OID.

○ **Focal joint space loss is typically encountered in which non-inflammatory arthropathy?**

Osteoarthritis.

○ **Osteoarthritic changes of the lateral column joints are most frequently associated with what 2 underlying local (non-systemic) pathologies?**

Tarsal coalition and trauma.

○ **Heel pad thickening has been associated with chronic usage of which drug?**

Dilantin.

○ **The Wimberger ring (halo epiphysis) is classically encountered with which disorder?**

Barlow's disease or scurvy.

○ **Phase I Paget's disease manifests radiographically with?**

Advancing osteolysis with a well-defined zone of transition.

○ **A rare osteosclerotic disorder characterized by a failure of osteoclastic resorption and the radiographic presence of "bones within bones"?**

Osteopetrosis.

○ **Two drugs most frequently associated with avascular necrosis when used on a chronic basis?**

Steroids, alcohol (also occasionally indomethacin and phenylbutazone).

○ **Of scurvy, congenital syphilis, rickets, osteomalacia, and congenital rubella, the disorder most frequently associated with pseudofractures?**

Osteomalacia.

○ **Two disorders routinely associated with ballooning of the epiphyses?**

Juvenile RA/juvenile chronic arthritis and hemophilic arthropathy.

○ **A fracture of the distal tibia in children classically described as a combination of the juvenile Tillaux fracture and a coronal plane Salter-Harris II?**

Juvenile triplane fracture of the tibia.

○ **Name two true arthropathies known to affect the ankle joint which are associated with very late or absent joint space loss.**

Chronic gouty arthritis, synovial chondromatosis, haemophilic arthropathy, juvenile chronic arthritis, and pigmented villonodular synovitis (PVNS).

○   **List 2 radiographic features characteristic of Stage I Eichenholz classification for diabetic Charcot joint arthropathy.**

Fine periarticular fragmentation with subluxation.

○   **The radiographic presence of lysis in osteomyelitis complicating the diabetic foot is not, in of itself, a criterion to amputate because?**

Significant bony lysis generally occurs with an intact vascular supply.

○   **On an anterior-posterior pedal radiograph, you notice pseudoforaminae formation on almost all of the distal phalanges. Although sometimes encountered as a normal variant, what systemic disorder remains high in the list of differentials?**

Acromegaly.

○   **Name two radiographic features distinguishing pyogenic septic arthritis from tuberculous septic arthritis.**

TB - much slower progression of disease with development of osteoporosis prior to erosions. Erosions typically start marginal (non-contact) and proceed to central space late. Late loss of joint space with endstage fibrous ankylosis typical.

○   **When evaluating standard ankle AP and mortise radiographs for a patient who has chronic ankle pain secondary to an old ankle sprain, you notice a possible distal fibular colliculus avulsion fragment. What is the simplest way to distinguish this from a normal os subfibulare?**

Inversion stress ankle studies - the os subfibulare will not displace.

○   **A processes x-ray film, when held up to a light source, has been darkened to the degree that only 1 out of every 100 photons of incident light is transmitted (1% transmittance) through the film. The optical film density (OD) is therefore?**

2.0.

○   **Name two relatively non-aggressive or benign bone tumors routinely found in the epiphyses.**

Chondroblastomas and giant cell tumors.

○   **An epiphyseal osteochondroma most frequently located in the medial ankle?**

Dysplasia epiphysealis hemimelica (or Trevor's disease).

○   **The radiographic hallmark of chronic osteomyelitis?**

Sequestered bone.

○   **It has been noted that adult-onset RA involving the midfoot joints has a different set of radiographic features than when the classic MPJ levels are involved. Specifically, what are two major differences noted in the midfoot?**

Lacks significant marginal erosions and there is a predilection for endstage bony ankylosis. In addition, subchondral sclerosis is typical with joint space loss and secondary osteoarthritic changes may be seen.

○ **When CT scans of the foot are ordered, which plane generally can not be directly imaged**

Sagittal plane.

○ **Calcium pyrophosphate deposition disease seems to have a predilection for which pedal joint?**

Talocalcaneonavicular joint.

○ **In comparing the radiographic features of wear & tear versus secondary osteoarthritis, what is the key radiographic difference at virtually any involved pedal location?**

Early concentric joint space loss is typical in secondary osteoarthritis.

○ **The lateral radiographs of a patient with heel pain demonstrate fine, linear calcifications of the plantar fascial and Achilles tendon attachment sites into the calcaneus. You suspect underlying CPPD. Name two extra-pedal screening sites for chondrocalcinosis and therefore confirmation.**

Knee, symphysis pubis, wrist.

○ **MR evaluation of an ankle for suspected Achilles tendon rupture reveals a well-defined lesion in the belly of the soleus muscle demonstrating shortening of both the T1 & T2 relaxation times. The lesion is most likely?**

Intramuscular lipoma.

○ **In standard spin-echo imaging, what is the general trend in relaxation times for structures that are either infected or inflamed?**

T1 & T2 relaxation times are lengthened.

○ **When viewing an MR scan of the foot, a particular pathologic infiltrate lengthens both the T1 & T2 relaxation times of that tissue. What is the predicted end result upon the actual signal intensities on both T1- and T2-weighted images?**

The pathologic infiltrate will appear darker on T1-weighted images and brighter on T2-weighted images.

○ **List 2 major radiographic differences between gouty tophi and rheumatoid nodules.**

Rheumatoid nodules do not calcify and are rarely associated with underlying bony destruction.

○ **In standard spin-echo imaging, an image with a long TE and a long TR is?**

T2-weighted.

○ **In standard spin-echo imaging, an image with a short TE and a long TR is?**

Balanced or proton density.

○ **A middle age obese female patient with sudden onset of arch pain undergoes MR evaluation only to reveal a Stage II posterior tibial tendon rupture. What are the MR findings in support of this?**

Decreased caliber of the tendon, equal to or smaller than the diameter of the adjacent FDL tendon. Complete rupture is not apparent.

○   **The "fallen-fragment" sign is virtually pathognomic for which lesion?**

Simple bone cyst.

○   **True osteochondromas are virtually never found in:**

Epiphyses.

○   **An endocrine disorder which typically manifests irregular "stippled" epiphyses?**

Cretinism.

○   **Wimberger's classic radiographic sign of congenital syphilis is?**

Bilateral symmetric destruction of the proximal medial tibial metaphyses.

○   **A patient presents with focal shortening of some of the small tubular foot bones, bone infarcts and coarsened trabecular patterns. Axial studies demonstrate "H" vertebrae. A most likely diagnosis is?**

Sickle-cell disease.

○   **Although bone scans are generally nonspecific, a pattern of juxta-articular uptake involving all of the joints of a symptomatic extremity is strongly suggestive (up to 90% specific) of?**

Reflex sympathetic dystrophy.

○   **On a weight-bearing lateral radiograph, the sum total of the calcaneal inclination and talar declination angles will always equal?**

The lateral talocalcaneal angle.

○   **On the lateral pedal radiograph, the Meary-Tomeno line passes substantially inferior to the 1st metatarsal head. This foot is most likely**

Pronated or flat.

○   **Which two radiographic features of secondary hyperparathyroidism (HPT) are infrequently encountered in the picture of primary HPT?**

Osteosclerosis and periostitis.

○   **Name one pediatric disorder whose radiographic picture is characterized by longitudinal sclerotic lines in long bones?**

Osteopatha striata (Voorhoeve's disease), congenital rubella (celery stick appearance), and hypophosphatasia.

○   **The periarticular erosive changes in adult RA generally stay small. However, erosions 5.0 mm or greater are not uncommonly encountered at what pedal site?**

5th metatarsophalangeal joint.

❑   **The development of silver halide crystals on the film by a process other than exposure to x-rays is known as?**

Film fog.

❑   **Polyostotic fibrous dysplasia is routinely included in the differential diagnosis of diffusely "ballooned" tubular bones of the foot. Individual lesions of polyostotic and monostotic fibrous dysplasia, however, tend to differ. List two key differences**

Monostotic lesions tend to be geographic type B lesions with well-defined, sclerotic margins whereas polyostotic lesions gradually blend with normal bone.
Monostotic lesions initially tend to expand the cortex eccentrically whereas polyostotic lesions tend to display fusiform expansion.
Gross bending deformities and fractures more common in polyostotic disease.
"Ground glass" appearance more common in polyostotic disease.

❑   **Acrolysis of the mid-portions of multiple distal phalanges in a bilateral symmetric pattern should suggest one of 3 conditions:**

Hyperparathyroidism, acrolysis of Hajdu & Cheny, and PVC overexposure (tank cleaners).

❑   **On an A-P radiograph of a hallux valgus deformity, you notice that PASA + DASA = HA Geometrically, what can be said about the joint?**

The joint must be congruous.

❑   **A patient presents with recent onset of heel pain. Lateral pedal radiographic findings demonstrate large irregular heel spurs suggestive of an underlying systemic enthesopathy. Significant bony sclerosis is noted. Of hypoparathyroidism, DISH, fluorosis, and seronegative arthritis, which is least likely?**

DISH.

❑   **The radiographic and clinical features of mixed connective tissue disease represent overlap of what four disorders?**

Scleroderma, systemic lupus, dermatomyositis, and rheumatoid arthritis.

❑   **Methods of reducing scatter radiation include frugal collimation, employing grids, shortened exposure times, going from single screen to double screens, and decreasing the kilovoltage. Two of these techniques will increase patient dosage - which two?**

Decreasing kilovoltage and employing grids.

❑   **Film badges and thermoluminescent dosimeters are standard means whereby the quantity of radiation received by an occupational worker in your office can be grossly determined. Not everyone, however, requires monitoring. Who should be monitored?**

Personnel monitoring is required when there is any likelihood that an individual will receive more than one quarter of the dose limit.

❑   **With respect to the most current dose limits (based upon the 1993 NCRP report) for occupational exposure to radiation, what is the annual limit for whole body radiation?**

50 mSv (5000 mrem or 5.0 rem).

○   **With respect to the most current dose limits (based upon the 1993 NCRP report) for occupational exposure to radiation, what is the annual limit for radiation to the skin, hands or feet?**

500 mSv (50,000 mrem or 50 rem).

○   **With respect to the most current dose limits (based upon the 1993 NCRP report) for occupational exposure to radiation, how is the cumulative or lifetime limit for whole body radiation determined?**

Age x 1.0 rem (10 mSv x age).

RHEUMATOLOGY

○   **Systemic Sclerosis (scleroderma) may be divided into two major subsets: Diffuse Cutaneous Systemic Sclerosis and Limited Cutaneous Systemic Sclerosis. The group with Limited Cutaneous Systemic Sclerosis is also known as?**

The CREST variant.

○   **What do the letters CREST, stand for in this variant?**

Calcinosis, Raynaud's, Esophagitis, Sclerodactyly, and Telangiectasias.

○   **Is Nailfold Capillary Microscopy a useful tool in the diagnosis of systemic sclerosis?**

Yes, the observation of capillary dilation, capillary destruction, and capillary hemorrhage are the positive findings.

○   **Can psoriatic arthritis precede the development of psoriatic skin lesions?**

Yes, this happens in approximately 15-20% of cases of psoriatic arthritis.

○   **Do all patients with psoriasis develop psoriatic arthritis?**

No, only about 6-20% of patients with psoriasis will develop psoriatic arthritis. It usually follows months to years of skin involvement but occasionally develops simultaneously.

○   **What are the patterns of involvement of psoriasis in the nails?**

Pitting, transverse or longitudinal ridging, "oil droplet" discoloration, subungual hyperkeratosis, and onycholysis.

○   **Which are the sero-negative arthritides?**

Reiter's disease, Psoriatic arthritis, Ankylosing Spondylitis, and the Arthritis of Inflammatory Bowel Disease (Crohn's disease and Ulcerative Colitis).

○   **The plaques of psoriasis contain large counts of which bacteria?**

Streptococcus, particularly group A.

○   **What are the Criteria for the Classification of Rheumatoid Arthritis according to the American Rheumatology Association?**

1. Morning stiffness (for at least 6 weeks).
2. Arthritis of 3 or more joint areas (for at least 6 weeks).
3. Arthritis of hand joints (for at least 6 weeks).
4. Symmetric arthritis (for at least 6 weeks).
5. Rheumatoid nodules.
6. Serum rheumatoid factor.
7. Radiographic changes.
For classification purposes, a patient has RA if they satisfy at least 4 of these 7 criteria.

○   **In reference to rheumatology, what is a DMARD ?**

"Disease Modifying Antirheumatic Drug." Also known as slow acting antirheumatic drugs. These drugs are thought to favorably modify the progression of rheumatoid arthritis as measured by radiographic evidence such as joint erosions or joint destruction.

○   **What are the factors predisposing to acute bacterial infections in a joint?**

Underlying joint disease such as rheumatoid arthritis, osteoarthritis, diabetes mellitus, immunosuppressive therapy, advanced age, alcoholism, and prosthesis or other foreign body in the joint.

○   **What is the most frequent cause of septic arthritis in immunocompetent individuals younger than 40 years of age?**

Disseminated gonococcal infection.

○   **What is the classic triad seen in disseminated gonococcal infection?**

Migratory tenosynovitis, vesiculopustular skin lesions, and oligoarthralgia. This triad only occurs in about 50% of patients however.

○   **What is the most urgent reason for performing synovial fluid analysis?**

To rule out infectious arthritis.

○   **What are the characteristics of normal synovial fluid?**

Normal synovial joint fluid is clear (transparent), the color ranges from colorless to straw colored, it is highly viscous, with less than 200 WBC/mm^3 of which less than 25% are PMN's. It contains no bacteria, no crystals and the glucose level is nearly equal to that of blood.

○   **What are the characteristics of an "inflammatory" joint fluid?**

"Inflammatory" joint fluid is usually translucent or opaque. The color ranges from a yellowish to yellowish-green. It has decreased viscosity, with greater than 2,000 WBC/mm^3 of which greater than 50% are PMN's. It may contain bacteria or crystals depending on the etiology of the inflammation.

○   **What is the proliferating synovium seen in rheumatoid arthritis?**

Pannus.

○   **What is the course of joint destruction seen in rheumatoid arthritis?**

Erosion of juxta-articular bone around the margins of the pannus and invasion of subchondral tissue by the pannus.

○   **What is the serious complication seen in the cervical spine in rheumatoid patients?**

Progressive erosion of the cervical vertebrae leading to atlantoaxial subluxation which can give rise to spinal cord compression.

○   **Behind the knee, enlargement of the semimembranous bursa into the popliteal space is referred to as:**

Baker's cyst. These sometimes rupture and mimic symptoms of acute thrombophlebitis.

❍ **What is the most common clinical lesion of rheumatoid arthritis seen in the heel?**

Retrocalcaneal bursitis.

❍ **High titers of rheumatoid factor are most commonly seen in the presence of ?**

Rheumatoid nodules.

❍ **What is the significance of very high titers of rheumatoid factor?**

High titers are generally associated with a more generalized systemic disease process and a more erosive, destructive arthritic process.

❍ **What is the histology of a rheumatoid nodule?**

Fibrinoid necrosis within a palisade of radially elongated connective tissue cells that form a corona around the necrosis. This is enclosed by an outer layer of granulation tissue consisting of chronic inflammatory cells, mostly lymphocytes and plasma cells.

❍ **What are the nonarticular manifestations of rheumatoid arthritis?**

Subcutaneous nodules, vasculitis, easy bruising, pericarditis, rarely pericardial tamponade, myocarditis, coronary arteritis, valvular insufficiency, conduction abnormalities, occasionally myocardial infarct, pleuritis, pleural effusion, interstitial fibrosis, inflammatory cell infiltrate of the lung, neuropathy, nerve compression, Sjögren's syndrome, episcleritis, scleromalacia perforans, Felty's syndrome, anemia, thrombocytopenia, leukopenia.

❍ **What are the Criteria for the Classification of Systemic Lupus Erythematosus according to the American Rheumatology Association?**

1. Malar rash.
2. Discoid rash.
3. Photosensitivity (by history or physician observed).
4. Oral ulcers (or nasopharyngeal – observed by a physician).
5. Arthritis (nonerosive involving 2 or more joints).
6. Serositis (pleuritis or pericarditis).
7. Renal disorder (proteinuria or cellular casts).
8. Neurologic disorder (seizures or psychosis).
9. Hematologic disorder (hemolytic anemia, or leukopenia, or lymphopenia, or thrombocytopenia).
10. Immunologic disorder (pos. LE cell prep., or anti-DNA, or anti-Sm or false positive serologic test for syphilis confirmed by FTA).
11. Antinuclear antibody.
For classification purposes, a patient has Lupus if they satisfy at least 4 or more of these 11 criteria serially or simultaneously.

❍ **What are Lupus Anticoagulants?**

Paradoxically named blood coagulation inhibitors, which are associated with thrombosis, not with hemorrhage. They are found in Lupus as well as other conditions. Anticardiolipin antibodies and Lupus anticoagulants are both antiphospholipid antibodies. The thrombotic manifestations, in addition to DVT and pulmonary emboli, may involve retinal vasculature, renal veins, coronary or mesenteric vessels and large peripheral arteries.

❍ **Which drug is the most frequent cause of a drug induced Lupus syndrome?**

Procainamide. Other drugs which have been reported to cause Lupus like syndromes include hydralazine, hydantoin anticonvulsants, isoniazid, alpha methyldopa, propylthiouracil, methimazole, quinidine and the sulfonamides as well as penicillin.

O   **What is the standard screening test for SLE?**

The fluorescent antinuclear antibody (ANA) test.

O   **Localized scleroderma, which begins with one or more areas of erythematous or violaceous discoloration of skin, which evolve to become sclerotic and waxy is referred to as:**

Morphea.

O   **What are the common manifestations of cutaneous involvement in systemic vasculitis?**

Cutaneous clinical manifestations include palpable purpura, ulcerations, livedo reticularis, and digital tip infarcts.

O   **What is Churg-Strauss Syndrome?**

Allergic granulomatosis and angiitis. It can be diagnosed on the basis of a history of asthma or allergic rhinitis, peripheral eosinophilia, and the development of a systemic vasculitis.

O   **What is Henoch-Schönlein Purpura?**

A disorder characterized by nonthrombocytopenic purpura, abdominal complaints, arthralgias, and renal involvement. It is also known as anaphylactoid or allergic purpura and usually occurs in children or young adults. Usually the first manifestation is palpable purpura of the lower extremities.

O   **What is the characteristic pathology of Goodpasture's Syndrome?**

Glomerulonephritis and pulmonary hemorrhage.

O   **What are cryoglobulins?**

Immunoglobulin molecules that have the unusual property of reversibly precipitating at low temperatures.

O   **What are the clinical manifestations of cryoglobulinemia?**

Monoclonal or mixed cryoglobulins cause vascular occlusive problems such as Raynaud's phenomena, cutaneous ulcers, and gangrene of fingers and toes, and cold-induced urticaria or arthralgias, purpura, nephritis and neuropathy.

O   **What is the sicca complex?**

Diminished salivary gland and lacrimal gland secretions.

O   **What is the triad originally described as Sjögren's Syndrome?**

Dry eyes, dry mouth, and rheumatoid arthritis.

O   **Can other diseases replace RA as part of Sjögren's syndrome?**

Yes, other connective tissue diseases such as SLE, Systemic Sclerosis, or Polymyositis may be present in place of RA.

○   **What is the laboratory test used to measure lacrimal gland secretion?**

The Schirmer filter paper test.

○   **An arthritis caused by the spirochete Borrelia burgdorferi is transmitted by the Ixodes dammini tick. What is the name of this disease?**

Lyme disease.

○   **What disease often begins with the skin rash, erythema chronicum migrans?**

Lyme disease.

○   **The rheumatic disease characterized by progressive loss of articular cartilage and by reactive changes at the margins of the joints and in subchondral bone is?**

Osteoarthritis.

○   **Describe the common clinical manifestations of osteoarthritis.**

Slowly developing joint pain which is at first present with activity and relieved with rest but later in the disease may be present with minimal motion or even at rest. Joint stiffness is relatively short lived (less than 60 minutes) and localized. Joint enlargement with limitation of motion. Pain on passive motion and crepitus are common. Associated secondary synovitis is common.

○   **Osteoarthritis of the distal interphalangeal joints of the hands is referred to as?**

Heberden's nodes.

○   **What is the variant of osteoarthritis which involves primarily the distal or proximal interphalangeal joints of the hands and whose painful inflammatory episodes are associated with eventual joint deformity and ankylosis.**

Erosive inflammatory osteoarthritis.

○   **What is the significant radiographic finding of erosive inflammatory osteoarthritis which is generally not seen in primary osteoarthritis?**

Bony erosions.

○   **What are the typical diagnostic laboratory findings seen in primary osteoarthritis?**

There are none. Laboratory findings are helpful in excluding other diagnoses only.

○   **What is the etiology of neuropathic osteoarthropathy or Charcot joint?**

This is controversial. One theory is termed the *neurotraumatic* pathogenesis theory and states that joint changes are caused by repetitive trauma to an insensate joint. Joint fatigue develops, leading to subluxation, microfractures, and further compromise. The other theory, termed the *neurovascular or hypervascular* pathogenesis theory states that autonomic neuropathy results in an increase in the peripheral perfusion to the lower extremity. This, in turn, weakens the osseous structures by washing out bone minerals, which leads to increases susceptibility to fractures. Many feel that the true pathogenesis is actually a combination of both processes.

O   **What is the most common clinical presentation of a Charcot foot?**

The typical patient is a diabetic (or has some other cause of neuropathy) with sensory neuropathy, and autonomic vasomotor neuropathy. Thus the patient will not appreciate the 5.07 Semmes-Weinstein monofilament. The pulses are usually bounding, with distended dorsal veins, and the foot is warm and very swollen. Findings depend on the Stage of the Neuroarthropathy.

> Stage I (Precollapse): perarticular swelling, joint effusion, normal foot alignment, normal radiographs except soft tissue swelling.
> Stage II (Collapse): increased swelling, increased local temperature, hypermobility, malalignment, fractures, fragmentation, and/or dislocation is seen on radiographs.
> Stage III (Healing): swelling and temperature decreases but this present, less hypermobility, hypertrophic bone formation and resorption of fine debris. Alignment unchanged.
> Stage IV (Arrest): no swelling, normal local temperature, decreased joint motion, alignment unchanged. Radiographs demonstrate consolidation of fragments and fractures.

O   **What is the most important differential diagnosis of an acute Charcot joint?**

Must rule out sepsis.

O   **How often is septic arthritis monoarticular?**

Septic arthritis is monoarticular 90% of the time and usually involves the large joints of the lower extremity. When it is polyarticular, it is usually in elderly patients with RA or who are receiving systemic corticosteroids.

O   **What is the most common bacteria causing nongonococcal septic arthritis?**

Staph. aureus accounts for 40% - 70% of purulent arthritis. Staph. aureus and staph. epidermidis are the most common organisms in prosthetic joint infections. Streptococcus is also not uncommonly seen in septic arthritis, approximately 25% of nongonococcal cases.

O   **What is the most common form of granulomatous arthritis?**

Joint sepsis with Mycobacterium tuberculosis is the most common form of granuomatous arthritis.

O   **Which is more common, Primary gout or Secondary gout?**

Primary gout accounts for 90% of cases.

O   **What is the name of an inherited case of "overproduction gout", characterized by hyperuricemia, mental retardation, self mutilation, choreoathetosis, and uric acid nephrolithiasis.**

Lesch-Nyhan syndrome.

O   **Lesch-Nyhan syndrome is the result of a total deficiency of what enzyme?**

Hypoxanthine guanine phosphoribosyl transferase (HGPRT).

O   **What are the stages of gout?**

Asymptomatic hyperuricemia, acute gouty arthritis, intercritical gout (which is the period between attacks), chronic tophaceous gout.

O   **List the Classification criteria for acute gouty arthritis.**

A. The presence of characteristic urate crystals in the joint fluid, or

B. A tophus proved to contain urate crystals by chemical means or polarized light microscopy, or

C. The presence of six of the following twelve clinical, laboratory, and x-ray phenomena listed below:

- More than one attack of acute arthritis
- Maximal inflammation developed within one day
- Attack of monoarticular arthritis
- Joint redness observed
- 1st MPJ painful or swollen
- Unilateral attack involving 1st MPJ
- Unilateral attack involving tarsal joint
- Suspected tophus
- Hyperuricemia
- Asymmetric swelling within a joint (roentgenogram)
- Subcortical cysts without erosions (roentgenogram)
- Negative culture of joint fluid for microorganisms during attack of joint inflammation

O **What is the most common cause of acute monoarticular or oligoarticular arthritis in the elderly?**

Acute pseudogout.

O **What joints are most commonly involved in pseudogout?**

Knee (58%), wrist (33%), ankle joint.

O **What is the most common joint involved in the foot?**

Talonavicular joint. Pseudogout involves the foot in only 5% of cases.

O **What are the differences in clinical presentation between gout and pseudogout?**

Patients with pseudogout tend to be older, and complain less of pain. Males and females are involved equally. Pseudogout does not respond as dramatically to colchicine as does gout.

O **Does the finding of chondrocalcinosis in the knee, wrist symphysis pubis, or any other joint require treatment for pseudogout?**

Most people with chondrocalcinosis remain asymptomatic. 60% of people over the age of 80 have chondrocalcinosis.

O **Does the finding of CPPD crystals in synovial fluid exclude the diagnosis of gout, RA, or infection?**

No! Pseudogout can coexist with these other diseases.

O **Chronic arthropathy of CPPD (calcium pyrophosphate dihydrate deposition disease) may overlap with osteoarthritis.   Examination may reveal limited ROM, crepitus, mild pain and synovitis. How can chronic pyrophosphate arthropathy be distinguished from osteoarthritis?**

By having more severe destruction of the joints and adjacent bone.

O **Gottron's papules and Gottron's sign are pathognomonic for what idiopathic inflammatory myopathy?**

Dermatomyositis.

O **What are Gottron's papules?**

These are violaceous, flat-topped papules overlying the dorsal surface of the interphalangeal joints of the hands. They can develop central atrophy, with telangiectasia and hypopigmentation. They occur in one third of patients with polymyositis. The cutaneous manifestations of dermatomyositis may precede, follow, or develop concomitantly with muscle involvement.

○   **What is Gottron's sign?**

Erythematous smooth or scaly patches, with or without associated edema, over the dorsal interphalangeal or metacarpophalangeal joints, elbows, knees, or medial malleoli. Gottron's sign is seem more commonly than Gottron's papules.

○   **Describe the facial rash sometimes seen in dermatomyositis.**

This is a heliotrope rash, which is dusky purple and occurs over the often edematous upper eyelids, especially along the edges. This is sometimes photosensitive. A similar rash may develop on the V-area of the neck, shoulders, and upper back.

○   **What is the clinical hallmark of polymyositis and dermatomyositis?**

Proximal muscle limb and neck weakness sometimes associated with muscle pain.

○   **What are the laboratory hallmarks of polymyositis and dermatomyositis?**

Elevated creatine phosphokinase (CPK), aldolase, lactic dehydrogenase, and the transaminases. A more or less characteristic EMG pattern is also seen. Myoglobulinemia and myoglobinuria are commonly present. Autoantibodies are present in most patients. These include anti-Jo-1, anti-RNP, anti-PM-Scl, anti-Ro, anti-La, and anti-Mi. Muscle biopsy is usually indicated to establish the diagnosis.

○   **Describe the clinical syndrome of Polymyalgia Rheumatica.**

This a relatively common syndrome which is characterized by severe aching and stiffness in the neck, shoulder girdle or pelvic girdle muscle areas that lasts for a month or longer if untreated. The stiffness is worse in the morning and after periods of rest. The syndrome is generally seen in patients over 50 years of age and women predominate 2:1. Systemic symptoms are present in many patients and include malaise, weight loss, and low grade fever.

○   **What laboratory finding is considered an important diagnostic feature of Polymyalgia Rheumatica?**

An elevated erythrocyte sedimentation rate to at least 40 or 50 mm in 1 hour. (Westergren).

○   **What are some synonyms for Giant Cell Arteritis?**

Temporal arteritis, cranial arteritis, and granulomatous arteritis.

○   **What is the dreaded complication of Temporal Arteritis?**

Blindness due to the narrowing of the ophthalmic or posterior ciliary arteries. Permanent vision loss is seen in 8-15% of patients.

○   **Can Temporal Arteritis affect the arteries of the lower extremities?**

Yes, although the vessels most commonly affected are branches of the arteries originating from the arch of the aorta.

O **What disease often presents with tenderness or enlargement of involved portions of the arteries of the head and neck?**

Temporal Arteritis.

O **What is the treatment for Polymyalgia Rheumatica?**

 Systemic steroids.

O **What is the treatment for Temporal Arteritis?**

Systemic steroids.

O **Unexplained proteinuria, peripheral neuropathy, enlargement of the tongue, cardiomegaly, intestinal malabsorption, bilateral carpal tunnel syndrome, or orthostatic hypotension should alert the clinician to the possible diagnosis of ?**

Primary Amyloidosis.

O **In Ankylosing Spondylitis, what is the difference in involved joint distribution between men and women?**

In men, AS is an arthritis of the sacroiliac joints, to a varying degree the rest of the spine, and to a lesser extent peripheral joints. Women are less likely to have progressive spinal disease. They tend to have more peripheral joint manifestations. This leads to the misdiagnosis of seronegative rheumatoid arthritis.

O **What is the pathognomonic test for Ankylosing Spondylitis?**

There is none. HLA-B27 is positive in 90-95% of patients. Sed. Rate may be elevated. Radiographic evidence of sacroiliitis is seen. AS is generally diagnosed on clinical grounds.

O **Which peripheral joints are most commonly involved in Ankylosing Spondylitis?**

Shoulders and hips. Peripheral joint involvement is seen in 20-30% of patients.

O **Where is enthesitis seen in the foot in Ankylosing Spondylitis?**

Achilles tendon insertion and the calcaneal plantar fascial insertion.

O **Do patients with Ankylosing Spondylitis develop eye problems (uveitis)?**

Up to 25% of patients will develop uveitis during their illness. It is more commonly seen in patients who are HLA-B27 positive, and have peripheral joint disease.

O **Why is Reiter's syndrome considered a reactive disease?**

Because it usually follows an infectious episode, either GI or GU (nongonococcal).

O **In terms of Reiter's syndrome, what is meant by the "complete syndrome?"**

The original description of Reiter's syndrome consisted of a triad of arthritis, urethritis, and conjunctivitis. Patients with these three components are said to have the complete syndrome.

O   **What are the cutaneous manifestations of Reiter's Syndrome?**

Circinate balanitis, and keratoderma blennorrhagicum. Superficial oral ulcers may also be seen in the mouth.

O   **What other skin disease is indistinguishable from keratoderma blennorrhagicum, macroscopically and microscopically?**

Pustular psoriasis.

O   **What is the most common location for keratoderma blennorrhagicum?**

The soles of the feet, but it can also be seen on the palms, the scrotum and elsewhere.

O   **What percentage of patients with Reiter's Syndrome will be HLA-B27 positive?**

80-90%

O   **Will treatment with antibiotics alter the course of patients with Reiter's Syndrome?**

No, there is no evidence for this.

O   **Describe the musculoskeletal findings in Reiter's Syndrome.**

Acute onset of an asymmetric polyarthritis or oligoarthritis involving the knees or ankles. Other joint involvement is less common. Dactylitis or sausage digits (fingers or toes) are seen. Tenderness and swelling at the tendo Achilles insertion and tenderness of the calcaneal insertion of the plantar fascia. Low back pain and/or sacroiliitis.

O   **What disease is associated with the term "Lover's heel?"**

Reiter's Syndrome.

O   **What percentage of the general white population will be HLA-B27 positive?**

About 6%.

O   **What percentage of patients with inflammatory bowel disease will develop peripheral arthritis?**

About 15-20%.

O   **Which peripheral joints are most often affected by inflammatory bowel disease?**

Knees and ankles.

O   **What percentage of patients with inflammatory bowel disease will develop sacroiliitis?**

About 20%.

O   **What percentage of patients with inflammatory bowel disease, and sacroiliitis will develop spondylitis?**

About 20%; this is about 4-5% of all patients with inflammatory bowel disease.

O   **What percentage of patients with inflammatory bowel disease, sacroiliitis, and spondylitis with be HLA-B27 positive?**

About half of them.

O   **Does the enteropathic spondylitis follow the course of the bowel disease?**

No.

O   **Carditis, acute polyarthritis, chorea, erythema marginatum and subcutaneous nodules are characteristic of what illness?**

Acute rheumatic fever.

O   **What is the most common etiology of acute rheumatic fever?**

A preceding beta-hemolytic streptococcal pharyngitis.

O   **A multisystem disorder of unknown etiology characterized histologically by the presence of noncaseating epithelioid cell granulomas in affected tissues is known as ?**

Sarcoidosis.

O   **What tissues are affected most commonly early in the course of sarcoidosis?**

Lung, skin, eyes.

O   **What is the most common rheumatic manifestation of sarcoidosis?**

Acute arthritis (15%).

O   **A form of sarcoidosis, in which the triad of bilateral hilar adenopathy, erythema nodosum, and arthritis is present, is known as?**

Löfgren's syndrome.

O   **Which joints are commonly affected by sarcoidosis?**

Ankles, knees, PIPJ's, wrists, and elbows.

O   **Patients with fibrositis complain of three major symptoms. What are they?**

Musculoskeletal pain, stiffness, and easy fatigability. Sleep disturbances are also a common feature.

O   **The hallmark of the examination of a fibrositis patient is the lack of objective findings in relation to the plethora of symptoms. What is the only abnormal finding?**

The presence of numerous discreet tender points, which should not be confused with trigger points.

O   **What is the difference between the tender points seen in fibrositis and the trigger points seen in myofascial pain syndromes?**

Palpation of a trigger point causes pain to be referred to a nearby regional site, whereas palpation of a tender point causes only local pain.

❍ **Clubbing of the digits in association with periostitis of the long bones should make one suspicious of what?**

Hypertrophic (pulmonary) osteoarthropathy (HOA). This is often associated with severe internal illness, often bronchogenic carcinoma.

❍ **The following radiographic criteria establish the diagnosis of what disease?**
- **Flowing calcification and ossification along the anterolateral aspect of at least four contiguous vertebral bodies.**
- **Relative preservation of intervertebral disc height**
- **Absence of intraarticular bony ankylosis of the sacroiliac and apophyseal joints**

Diffuse Idiopathic Skeletal Hyperostosis (DISH).

❍ **What is the Schober test?**

This tests the restriction of lumbar motion in patients with spondylitis. Two midline points, separated by 10 cm, are placed on the skin of the patient's lower back while standing. The first mark is at the level of the posterior superior iliac spines. The second 10 cm. above. The patient is then asked to bend forward in an attempt to touch the toes. Knees are kept straight. This should reverse the normal lumbar lordosis. As the skin over the lumbar area stretches, the two marks should now separate by at least 5 cm. to a total distance of 16-22 cm.

❍ **A benign disorder of unknown etiology which is characterized by the formation of multiple foci of metaplastic hyaline cartilage within the synovium is called?**

Synovial osteochondromatosis.

❍ **A benign disease of unknown etiology characterized by circumscribed or diffuse thickening of the synovial lining of joints, tendon sheaths, or bursae and the production of locally invasive, tumorlike growths is called?**

Pigmented Villonodular Synovitis.

❍ **What is the name of pigmented villonodular synovitis when it is manifested as an isolated, discrete lesion involving tendon sheath?**

Giant Cell Tumor of Tendon Sheath (or localized nodular tenosynovitis).

SOFT TISSUE, NAIL, AND DIGITAL TRAUMA

○ **Describe the Patzakis classification for zones of the plantar aspect of the foot.**

Zone 1 - extends from the neck to the metatarsals to the end of the digits.
Zone 2 - includes the area between the distal end of the calcaneus and the metatarsal necks.
Zone 3 - the area occupied by the calcaneus.
Zone 1 and 3 are associated with an increased incidence of osseous involvement and complications following a
     puncture wound.

○ **In a puncture wound with a retained foreign body, how long does it take an infection to manifest?**

Infection often manifests in 24 hours but may take three to four days.

○ **Why are structures such as intrinsic tendons, extrinsic tendons, intermetatarsal bursa, and MTPJ capsule of worry with puncture wounds?**

If a puncture wound extends to structures such as these, infection can be established easily due to their decreased vascularity and slower metabolic rate.

○ **Can glass be visualized on plain radiographs?**

Yes. Glass does not have to contain lead to be visualized. The size of the glass fragment is the limiting factor.

○ **What type of imaging study is best for detecting wood fragments?**

CT with use of narrow window.

○ **When does osteomyelitis become evident radiographically?**

10-14 days after establishment of bone infection. Tc-pp MDP bone scans demonstrate a focal uptake within 24 hours; however, they have low specificity. For better specificity, use a Tc-99 labeled leukocyte scan (HMPAO).

○ **How does osteomyelitis appear on MRI?**

T1 demonstrates decreased signal intensity.
T2 demonstrates increased signal intensity.

○ **What is the gold standard for diagnosis of osteomyelitis?**

Bone biopsy.

○ **What are the indications for incision and drainage following a puncture wound?**

Wound infection, presence of an abscess, and if a reactive foreign object is retained in the wound.

O   **What are the most common pathogens associated with soft tissue infections?**

Staphylococcus aureus, Staphylococcus epidermidis, and Streptococcus.

O   **What is the most common organism isolated from puncture wounds caused by cat and dog bites and first line treatment?**

Pasteurella multocida treated by Augmentin.

O   **What organism is most commonly isolated in osteomyelitis following a puncture wound?**

Pseudomonas aeruginosa.

O   **What is the most common site for osteomyelitis following puncture wound to the foot?**

The calcaneus.

O   **What is the most common object to cause a puncture wound?**

Nails are the most common at 98%. Other objects include wood, metal, and glass.

O   **What are some possible complications of puncture wounds?**

Soft tissue infection, osteomyelitis, foreign body granuloma, premature epiphyseal closure, joint degeneration, and residual deformity.

O   **How often is cellulitis seen after a puncture wound?**

8.4% of patients seen within the first 24 hours after injury, present with cellulitis within four days. If the patient is seen 1-7 days after injury, 57% develop cellulitis.

O   **What are the three classes of Pseudomonas infection in children described by Green and Bruno?**

Type I - early diagnosis and surgical drainage with antibiotic coverage results in complete healing.
Type II - diagnosis delayed 9-14 days. Debridement and antibiotics eradicate infection but patient may have
            residual bone or joint deformity.
Type III - diagnosis delayed over three weeks results in chronic infection with necessary bone resection.

O   **What are the goals of puncture wound treatment?**

Conversion of contaminated wound to a clean wound and prevention of tetanus.

O   **Tetanus prophylaxis is based on what four components?**

Wound care, tetanus toxoid, immune globulin, and antibiotics.

O   **How often should tetanus boosters be administered?**

For patients with an indeterminate number of toxoid injections, last injection was greater than one year and the wound is tetanus prone, administer the booster. If the wound is non-tetanus prone, a booster should be administered at intervals of five years.

O   **What is the most commonly encountered foreign body in the foot?**

A pin or needle.

O   **What are some possible complications of animal bites?**

Cellulitis, lymphangitis, abscesses, osteomyelitis, subcutaneous gas, meningitis, endocarditis, tularemia, and syphilis.

O   **Necrotic arachnidism is seen in what type of bite?**

Necrotic arachnidism is seen in brown recluse spider bites of the genus *Loxosceles*.
Necrotic arachnidism is described as severe necrotic tissue destruction. A blue-gray halo appears peri-puncture site which progresses to necrosis, eschar formation, and a large ulceration.

O   **What is the treatment for brown recluse spider bites?**

Treatment is controversial but may include intralesional and oral steroids, surgical debridement, and the use of dapsone.

O   **What is the difference between a low velocity and a high velocity projectile?**

Low velocity is ≤ 2000ft/second, high velocity is ≤ 2000ft/second

O   **According to the kinetic energy theory, what formula describes the amount of energy possessed by a projectile?**

$KE = 1/2\ mv^2$

O   **Describe the classification for shotgun wounds and name its developers.**

Sherman and Parrish described a classification for shotgun wounds.
     Type I - Penetrate subcutaneous tissue or deep fascia: Occur at distances greater than 7 yards.
     Type II Occur a 3-7 yards. Viscera, bones, and vascular system violated.
     Type III - Occur at less than 3 yards. Severe local destruction and loss of tissue.

O   **Describe Ordog's classification for gunshot wounds.**

Type 0 - No injury.
Type I - Blunt injury (nonpenetrating gunshot wound).
Type II - Graze injury (abrasion, injury to epidermis, superficial dermis).
Type III - Blast effect without missile penetration (bullet missed, blank ammo).
Type IV - Blast effect with missile penetration.
Type V - Penetrating. A - laceration through dermis, B - subcutaneous, C - all deep structures, D - body cavity, E - more than one body region.
Type VI - Perforating. A, B, C, D, E.
Type VII - Penetration with missile embolization.

O   **What are the basic tenants for simple low velocity missile wound care?**

Adequate nonoperative stabilization of fractures.
Adequate debridement of exposed necrotic tissue.
Cleansing of the wound with irrigation.
Closure without tension.
Wound observation for 48-72 hours.

❍   **What are the basic tenants for complex low velocity missile wound care?**

Cleansing with antiseptics/jet lavage.
Open reduction of fracture sites utilizing internal/external fixation.
Intravenous broad-spectrum antibiotics.
Daily wound observation and care until clinically uninfected and viable.
Primary versus delayed primary versus secondary closure.

❍   **What are the basic tenants of shotgun wound care?**

Arteriography.
Rapid debridement.
Sharp dissection.
Broad fasciotomy.
Pressure irrigation.
Tetanus prophylaxis.
Bony stabilization.
Vascular, neural, musculotendinous repair, including gastrocnemius flaps.
Delayed closure.
Antibiotic-impregnated materials to fill dead space.
Synthetic skin substitutes.
Frequent redebridement.
Closure/split-thickness skin graft at 7-10 days.

❍   **Generally, low velocity gunshot wounds are considered what type in Gustilo's classification?**

Type I.

❍   **What is lead intoxication called?**

Plumbism.

❍   **What is the antibiotic of choice for Type I gunshot wounds?**

Cephalosporin.

❍   **Is "Cavitation" associated with low or high velocity gunshot wounds?**

High velocity.

❍   **What are the factors, which determine the size and extent of damage produced by a projectile?**

The type of tissue the projectile penetrates, the bullet's composition, the bullet or bone fragmentation creating secondary missiles, and the amount of energy that the projectile dissipates in the tissue.

❍   **What is the largest organ in the body?**

The integumentary system is the largest organ in the body, comprising 15% of the total body weight.

❍   **Describe the classification for burn injury.**

First Degree - characterized by erythema without blister formation and are partial thickness (sunburns).
Second Degree - Are partial thickness but can be divided into superficial and deep. Superficial affect the deep layers of the epidermis but do not affect the basal cell layer and present with blister formation and pain. Deep

second degree burns involve mucc of the basal cell layer and my/may not have blister formation, may be dry and anesthetic.
Third Degree - Destruction of the full thickness of the skin and its appendages and are leathery, whitish to dark, and possible thrombosed vessels.

O   **What is used for fluid replacement for the first 24 hours after a burn and how much?**

Baxter's formula of 4ml of crystalloid per percent of total body surface area per kilogram of weight.

O   **Describe the stages of skin graft healing?**

Plasmatic.
Inosculation.
Revascularization.
Reinnervation.

O   **Describe the differentiation of split thickness skin grafts.**

Thin -- 0.008 - 0.012 inches in depth.
Intermediate - 0.012-0.016 inches in depth.
Thick - greater than 0.016 inches in depth.

O   **What are some possible complications of skin grafts that will cause a graft to fail?**

Seroma; Hematoma; Infection.

O   **What are phases of tendon healing?**

Impact - moment of injury, highlighted by the activation of the complement cascade.
Inflammatory phase - release of lactate and ascorbic acid to initiate fibroblastic activation in the low oxygen tension and acidic environment, stimulating collagen synthesis.
Proliferatory phase - increased collagen synthesis and revascularization.
Remodeling phase -continued collagen synthesis with organization of new tendon substance in a normal anatomical orientation.

O   **What are the Stages of tendon healing?**

The stages of tendon healing are based on chronology and are described according to weeks one through four, three months, and four months. During the first week following the initial injury the ruptured ends of the tendon become joined by a fibroblastic splint through a jelly-like bridge of serous and granulation tissue. Paratenon vascularity increases and collagen proliferates during the second week and the gap between ruptured ends is bridged in ten to fourteen days. The third week is noted to have collagen fibers beginning to coalesce and align longitudinally giving moderate strength to the tendon with reduction in edema and vascularity in the following week. At three months post-injury, there is noted small collagen bundle formation with anatomic orientation followed by larger collagen bundle formation (normal tendon) at four months.

O   **What is the Seddon classification?**

The Seddon classification describes nerve injury.

Neurapraxia - A conduction deficit without axonal destruction. Contusion or mild compression to a peripheral nerve.
Axonotmesis - Axonal disruption without destruction of the endoneurial tubes.

Neurotemesis – The axon and the connective tissue are lacerated and the ends are not realigned. Wallerian degeneration takes place.

○ **What is the Sunderland Classification?**

The Sunderland Classification also describes nerve injury.
First degree - Corresponds to neuropraxia and is a conduction deficit without axonal degeneration.
Second degree - Corresponds to axonotmesis and is axonal disruption without endoneurial disruption.
Third degree - Is a form or axonotmesis and neurotmesis and involves sectioning the axons with disruption of endoneurial tubes.
Fourth degree - Consists of physical disruption of the fascicles and perineurium with an intact epineurium.
Fifth degree - True neurotmesis or complete physical disruption of the nerve trunk.

○ **Who classified injuries about the nail? Describe them.**

Rosenthal classified these injuries and divided them into zones. Zone 1 involved injuries to the bony phalanx, zone 2 involves injuries distal to the lunula, and zone 3 involves injures proximal to the distal end of the lunula: Rosenthal suggested treatment options based on the zone of injury.

○ **What is a "clean" or "tidy" wound?**

Clean wounds involve minimal soft tissue damage or contamination and do not require extensive debridement prior to closure. Clean wounds are unlikely to become infected.

○ **What is the number of organisms per gram of tissue that define infection of soft tissue?**

10^5.

○ **What is the number of organisms per gram of tissue that define infection of bone?**

10^6.

○ **What is the number of organisms per gram of tissue that define infection of soft tissue or bone when a foreign body is present?**

10^2.

○ **What are the stages of wound healing and the events associated with each stage?**

Substrate (lag) phase begins at injury and lasts until about day 3 or 4. During this phase, there is formation of a platelet-fibrin plug and PMNs are the predominant white cell. The second phase is the proliferation phase, which lasts from day 3 or 4 to about day 21. This stage is characterized by fibroblasts that lay down collagen, new vessels and fibers that cross the defect, the presence of myofibroblasts ("surgeon's cells") which have a contractile capability. The predominant white cell in the proliferation phase is the macrophage. The final phase of wound healing is the remodeling phase, which lasts from about day 21 up to a year. During this phase, collagen fibers are realigned parallel to the resting skin tension lines.

○ **Why are extreme dorsiflexion injuries of the digits especially worrisome with children?**

Extreme hyperflexion injuries in children can traumatically avulse the distal growth plate and produce a compound fracture.

○ **What are some radiographic signs that can differentiate a bipartite sesamoid from a fractured sesamoid?**

The presence of irregular jagged edges between fragments as well as interrupted peripheral cortices is a good indicator. If a fracture is present the fragments if placed together, should resemble the size of a normal sesamoid. Conversely, if the sesamoid is bipartite, placing the fragments together would result in a larger than normal sesamoid.

○ **What is the sequela of removing an injured tibial sesamoid?**

Hallus valgus deformity.

○ **What adjunctive procedures should be considered when an injured tibial sesamoid is removed?**

Medial capsulorrhaphy and abductor hallucis tendon advancement will help to prevent a hallux valgus deformity.

○ **What is the most common fracture orientation in a lesser digit?**

Closed spiral oblique fracture.

○ **What is the easiest way to close reduce a digital fracture?**

Chinese finger trap apparatus.

○ **Why is the area around the ankle prone to the formation of fracture blisters?**

The area around the ankle is characterized by flatter epidermal papillae, sparse subcutaneous tissue, extensive arborizing veins, and lack of epidermal anchoring structures such as hair follicles and sweat glands.

○ **What locations other than the foot are prone to fracture blister formation?**

Elbow, foot, and distal tibia.

○ **What are the two types of fracture blisters?**

Clear (serous) fracture blisters are more prevalent while hemorrhagic blisters are thought to represent a more severe injury.

○ **Is the fluid in a fracture blister sterile?**

Yes.

○ **Between what two skin layers do fracture blisters form:**

Fracture blisters form at the dermal-epidermal junction.

○ **Histologically, a fracture blisters is very similar to what type of burn.**

Second-degree thermal burns.

○ **What type of internal fixation is best suited when crossing the physis in a digit?**

Smooth K-wires.

○ **What name is given to an osteochondrosis of the base of the phalanges?**

Thiemann osteochondroses.

○　**What measures can be taken to prevent the formation of fracture blisters?**

Elevation, ice, compressive dressings, and early ORIF.

○　**What are the two broad categories of compartment syndrome etiology?**

Those that cause an increase in compartment content and those that decrease compartment size.

○　**What is the most common etiology of compartment syndrome?**

Fracture.

○　**What are the five P's that describe the symptoms of compartment syndrome?**

Pain out of proportion, parestheslas, paralysis, pulselessness, and pallor.

○　**How many compartments are present in the foot?　Name them.**

There are four compartments in the foot: medial, lateral, central, and interosseous.

○　**What percentage of nail plate should be involved with subungual hematoma before the nail plate is avulsed and the nail bed is inspected for lacerations?**

≤ 25% of the nail plate.　Any lacerations should be repaired with fine suture.

○　**What is the greatest predisposing factor for the development of an infection following a puncture wound to the bottom of the foot?**

Retained foreign body.

○　**What percentage of puncture wounds to the bottom of the foot develop complications?**

10%.

○　**What percentage of complications, following puncture wounds to the bottom of the foot, develop osteomyelitis?**

≤ 2%.

○　**Under what circumstances is the use of tetanus immune globulin considered following a puncture wound to the foot?**

In a case where basic active immunity has not been attained, or where is has been attained but is greater than 10 years old with no boosters given since then, and the wound is very dirty and tetanus prone.

○　**In terms of trauma, what does the "Golden Period" refer to?**

The first 6-8 hours after an injury before significant contamination develops.

SPORTS MEDICINE

❍ **Blisters are generally the result of _____ stress.**

Shear/frictional.

❍ **List the mechanical causes of blisters.**

Wet socks.
Seams in shoegear/socks.
Poor fit of shoegear allowing sliding.
Wrinkes in socks.
Defects in sock liner of shoe or friction at orthotic edges.
Gait abnormalities which allow anterior/posterior shear/friction or medial/lateral shear/friction.

❍ **"Tennis toe" could best be described as _____.**

A subunqual hematoma.

❍ **What is the mechanism behind the development of "tennis toe?"**

Tennis toes results from the free end of the toenail catching in the toebox as the foot slides forward in the shoe, ie. low toe box, or long nail, or distal phalanx extensus, or foot sliding forward for various reasons.

❍ **In acute "hyperflexion" injuries of the hallux in athletes, which soft tissue structures would be most likely to be injured?**

Dorsal capsular structures, EHL tendon which may also produce an avulsion injury at the EHL tendon insertion into the dorsal aspect of the distal phalanx.

❍ **The mechanism of "turf toe" generally involve which forces?**

Axial compression and dorsiflexion at the 1st metatarsophalangeal joint.

❍ **What are some common associated physical findings with hallux limitus in athletes may include?**

Increases hallux abductus interphalangeus angle, hyperextension of the hallux IPJ, keratoma under the IPJ of the hallux, dystrophic hallux nail from catching in the toebox, subungual exostosis due to dorsal distal phalangeal pressure (secondary to hyperextension at the IPJ).

❍ **List 3 methods of conservative treatment for hallux limitus/rigidus which can be used in athletes.**

Morton's extension.
Stiffen the sole of the shoe or select a running shoe with a stiffer sole.
Choose a shoe with more of a "rocker bottom."

❍ **The common mechanical denominator in functional hallux limitus is____.**

Dorsiflexion, elevation of the 1st ray (metatarsus primus elevatus) with resulting dorsal 1st MPJ jamming and eventual joint destruction and bony proliferation.

○   **Where is the most common location of metatarsal stress fracture occurring in the central rays?**

Distal metaphyseal-diaphyseal junction.

○   **A common mechanical factor in the development of abductor hallucis muscle strain occurring in a runner may be _____.**

Hypermobility of the 1st ray requiring the abductor hallucis to overwork in attempt to try to stabilize the 1st ray on the ground/supporting surface.

○   **In acute hyperextension injuries of the 1st MPJ, which structures of the 1st MPJ are most likely to be injured?**

Plantar 1st MPJ capsular sprain/rupture, dorsal 1st MPJ joint jamming (base of proximal phalanx, head of 1st met), possible avulsion fracture of sesamoids.

○   **List 4 mechanical etiologies of sesamoiditis as occurs in athletes.**

Plantarflexed 1st ray.
Excessive STJ pronation with 1st ray dorsiflexion and eversion, exposing tibial sesamoid.
Equinus, uncompensated, partially compensated.
Forefoot contact activities.
Foot type, i.e. Rigid cavus.

○   **The most common fracture types involving the sesamoids in athletes are:**

Avulsion and compression.

○   **The most common cause of hallucal sesamoid fracture in athletes involves _____:**

Forceful landing on the forefoot with the hallux dorsiflexed, tensing the sesamoid apparatus, either "exposing" the sesamoids to compression injury or increasing tension on the sesamoids resulting in avulsion.

○   **List the causes of neuroma (perineural fibroma) seen in athletes.**

Enlarged metatarsal head; piling of metatarsal heads (ie supinated foot); excessive pronation with dorsiflexion, eversion and abduction of the forefoot against the lateral side of the shoe resulting in crowding of the metatarsal heads; dorsiflexed digits with an altered MPJ axis of rotation; depressed metatarsal heads (unequal levels); decreased forefoot cushion (shoes or fat pad); tight shoes in forefoot.

○   **List the biomechanical/structural defects, which may result in a Navicular stress fracture.**

Abnormal spring ligament function.
Abnormal posterior tibial tendon function.
Excessive subtalar and midtarsal joint pronation.
Short 1st metatarsal, long 2nd metatarsal.
Pes planus.
Navicular compression between talus and cuneiforms.

○   **What is the most common location and orientation for Navicular stress fracture is?**

In the central 1/3rd (middle 1/3rd) of the Navicular, oriented on the sagittal plane beginning at the Talonavicular joint, extending distally.

○ **What is the basic pathomechanical factor leading to the development of a Navicular stress fracture?**

There is a retrograde force back through the 2nd metatarsal to the intermediate cuneiform, to the central 1/3 of the Navicular. The Navicular, as the "keystone" of the arch is impinged between the forefoot distally and the Talus proximally, focusing stress on the Navicular, resulting in stress fracture.

○ **Describe the appearance of a Navicular stress fracture as would be seen on MRI.**

Decreased signal intensity in the Navicular (central) on T1 weighted images and increased signal intensity on T2 and STIR due to inflammatory edema.

○ **What is the most important treatment concept in Navicular stress fracture is?**

The patient should be non-weight bearing initially whether casted or surgically fixated.

○ **Os Tibiale Externum syndrome in athletes primarily involves dysfunction of which tendon?**

Posterior Tibial.

○ **List/describe shoe abnormalities or inadequacies which may contribute to Posterior Tibial tendonitis.**

Low durometer midsole.
Weak/short heel counter.
Lateral midsole flare.
Excessive sole flexibility.
Excessive room in heel area allowing excessive motion within shoe.

○ **List the biomechanical causes of anterior tibial tendonitis as may be seen in the athlete.**

Excessive STJ pronation with forefoot varus; equinus with weak anterior muscle (muscle imbalance); heavy heel strikers (rapid slapping of forefoot requiring tibialis anterior to work harder to decelerate the forefoot plantarflexion; tight tibialis anterior.

○ **Describe the mechanism of functional tarsal tunnel syndrome.**

Subtalar joint pronation/eversion produces traction on the posterior tibial nerve as well as retinacular tightening producing compression on the nerve.

○ **How are anterior process fractures of the calcaneus are classified?**

Rowe type IC fracture.

○ **What is the mechanism for anterior process calcaneal fractures occurring in athletes?**

Mechanical inversion stress with adduction of the forefoot/midfoot and a plantarflexed foot.

○ **List injuries which occur at or around the calcaneocuboid joint.**

Anterior process fracture of the calcaneus.
Bifurcate ligament sprain.
Rupture of the Extensor Digitorum Brevis muscle.
Cuboid Peroneal Syndrome (subluxed cuboid).
Compression fracture of the cuboid.

O   **Which portion of the bifurcate ligament is usually sprained?**

The calcaneocuboid portion.

O   **What are the differential diagnoses in an athlete complaining of heel pain?**

Heel Spur Syndrome; Plantar fasciitis; Calcaneal Stress fracture; Entrapment of 1st branch of the lateral plantar nerve (Baxter's nerve); Inferior calcaneal bursitis; Plantar fascial rupture; Calcaneal neoplasm; Fat Pad failure of the heel; Sero-negative/sero-positive arthritis; Secondary to acute trauma; Medial calcaneal nerve neuritis.

O   **Describe the typical appearance of a Calcaneal stress fracture.**

Sclerotic fracture line from anterior to the tubercles, extending posterior and superior, minimal to no periosteal reaction, blurring/blunting/disruption of the calcaneal trabeculae.   The fracture line is generally nearly perpendicular to the primary compression trabeculae, suggesting a "compression" factor and resulting in the sclerotic appearance of the fracture line.

O   **Calcaneal stress fractures are generally the result of which forces?**

Primarily compression, secondarily tension.

O   **Sever's disease could best be described as:**

A traction apophysitis.

O   **What are the common mechanical abnormalities associated with Sever's disease?**

Excessive pronation; Equinus.

O   **What are the pathomechanics which frequently lead to Haglund's deformity?**

Excessive motion of the rearfoot, primarily frontal, secondarily sagittal i.e. Due to rearfoot varus, forefoot valgus, plantarflexed 1st ray, etc.

O   **Radiographic findings seen in Haglunds deformity may include_____?**

High Calcaneal inclination angle; High Fowler and Phillip angle (>70 deg).
Posterior-superior calcaneus above parallel pitch lines.

O   **List 3 mechanical etiologies of Hallux Limitus/Rigidus.**

Hypermobile 1st ray (excessive STJ pronation, short 1st ray).
Dorsiflexed 1st ray.
(metatarsus primus elevatus, congenital or acquired).
Long 1st ray.
Trauma/DJD.

O   **List radiographic findings which may be seen with Hallux limitus.**

Asymmetrical joint space narrowing.
Marginal osteophytes.
Subchondral cysts.
Subchondral sclerosis.

Long or short 1st metatarsal.
Metatarsus primus elevatus.
Elevated HAI angle.

○   **What are the different varieties of Freiberg's Infraction?**

Type I – met head dies but heals by replacement.
Type II – head collapses but articular surface remains, +/- peripheral osteophytes.
Type III – head collapses with articular cartilage loosening, joint destroyed
Type IV – multiple heads involved.

○   **Describe the usual mechanisms in subluxed cuboid/cuboperoneal syndrome.**

Acute: ie. Post ankle sprain with the cuboid forced plantar and medial.
Chronic: Excessive lateral stress due to rearfoot varus, cavus foot, short limb compensations, equinus.
                 Chronic extrinsic stress, dorsiflexing forefoot/midfoot, ie. standing on rung of ladder for
                 prolonged periods.

○   **In subluxed cuboid syndrome, how is the Cuboid believed to move?**

Plantar and medial.

○   **Ligamentous structures most commonly involved in Sinus Tarsi Syndrome include:**

Interosseous talo-calcaneal ligament.
Cervical ligament.

○   **Soft tissue impingement of the ankle usually occurs in which areas?**

Anterolaterally and posteromedially.

○   **The mechanism of anterior bony impingement of the ankle generally involves:**

Forceful dorsiflexion jamming trauma, i.e. Jump and land forcing the foot in a rapid dorsiflexed position or rapid
explosive starts/push off with the foot in a dorsiflexed position.

○   **How does posterior leg muscle tone contribute to the development of anterior ankle impingement
syndrome?**

If low tone/strength in the posterior muscle group, rapid dorsiflexion of the ankle cannot be counteracted/decelerated
as effectively, resulting in anterior jamming.

○   **What is Ferkel's phenomenon?**

Soft tissue cause of anterolateral ankle impingement from scar/fibrosis and synovitis in anterolateral ankle gutter,
usually post-traumatic (post sprain).

○   **What is Basset's ligament?**

A slip of the anterior tibiofibular ligament, abnormally coursing down the lateral malleolus to the lateral border of
the talus, resulting in impingement syndrome of the ligament between the talus and fibula.

○   **What is the mechanism involved in posterior bony impingement of the ankle?**

The posterior tubercle, primarily posterolateral tubercle/process (Stieda's Process) becomes impinged between the posterior lip of the tibia and the superior surface of the calcaneus at the posterior edge of the posterior subtalar joint facet when the ankle is plantarflexed.

○   **Soft tissue posterior ankle impingement often involves which structures?**

Flexor Hallucis Longus tendon, posterior capsule and synovium.

○   **What classification system is used in osteochondral fractures of the Talar dome and how is the fracture staged?**

Berndt and Harty
> Stage I – chondral and subchondral compression.
> Stage II – incomplete fracture through subchondral zone but remains attached to talus.
> Stage III – complete fracture but fracture fragment remains in its crater.
> Stage IV – complete fracture which moves in its crater, flips or becomes loose within the joint.

○   **What are the typical differences between medial and lateral osteochondral fractures of the talus?**

Medial fractures tend to be deeper, more cup shaped, secondary to compression force. Lateral fractures tend to be shallower, more wafer shaped and generally secondary to shear forces.

○   **Lateral Talar process fractures in the athlete generally tend to be due to:**

The ankle is forcefully dorsiflexed and inverted with weight bearing forces becoming concentrated on the lateral process of the talus. The downward force of the talus is counteracted by the stable position of the calcaneus which transmits vertical ground reactive forces to the lateral talar process.

○   **What are the two most common mechanisms resulting in a posterior talar process fracture seen in the athlete?**

Forced dorsiflexion of the foot and ankle, avulsing the posterior process by ligamentous attachment; or extreme plantarflexion, ie. Sliding injury in baseball, where the posterior process is compressed between the posterior lip of the tibia superiorly driving downward and the posterior calcaneus inferiorly driving upward, shearing off the posterior process of the talus.

○   **The mechanism most commonly involved in traumatic subluxation of the peroneal tendons is:**

Forceful, resisted dorsiflexion and eversion of the ankle, i.e. Such as eversion/dorsiflexion of the foot against the rigidity of a ski boot.

○   **When the peroneal tendons traumatically dislocate, besides possible injury to the peroneal tendons, which other structures are injured allowing the subluxation/dislocation?**

The superior Peroneal retinaculum which may avulse a small strip of periosteum from the posterior surface of the lateral malleolus or produce an avulsion fracture from the posterior surface of the lateral malleolus which may be seen on an ankle mortise view or a medial oblique radiograph of the ankle.

○   **What are "shin splints?"**

An overuse, musculotendinous inflammatory condition of the shin region excluding injury to bone or of vascular etiology.

○   **What are the types of shin splints?**

Anterior, Posterior and Lateral depending on the muscle compartments or individual muscles involved.

O   **What are some mechanical precipitating factors leading to the development of shin splints?**

Biomechanical faults (depending on the fault, different muscles/groups are involved).
Muscle imbalances (weakness, tightness, improper ratios).
Early in training/beginning training/resuming training after a period of inactivity, etc.
Change in training schedule (ie. Increased effort = duration, stress, frequency, etc.).
Change in training methods.
Changes in surfaces.
Changes in shoegear.

O   **What are the different types of Posterior shin splints?**

Posterior tibial/Soleal shin splints which usually occur in the mid to lower Tibial along the posterior medial ridge, FHL shin splints which tend to be at the distal end of the Tibia along the posterior medial ridge and FDL shin splints which tend to be more proximal along the posterior medial ridge of the Tibia.

O   **How can running shoes contribute to the development of Posterior Tibial/Soleal shin splints?**

Factors in the running shoe which would allow the foot to excessively pronate would contribute to the development of Posterior Tibial/Soleal shin splints, i.e., wide flared heels (particularly lateral flare), low durometer midsole, weak counter, lack of medial shoe support, poor counter-midsole junction, etc.

O   **What are some mechanisms contributing to the development of anterior shin splints?**

Tight tibialis anterior (tends to be aggravated with downhill running and overstriding).
Tight posterior muscle group and weak tibialis anterior (AT needs to work harder to dorsiflex the foot/ankle and becomes overused. Tends to be worse with uphill running and understriding).
Overstress as a compensation for forefoot imbalance, i.e. forefoot varus where the tibialis anterior assists in decelerating the medial side of the forefoot to the ground.
Pathologically increased/high heel striker which forces rapid foot plantarflexion, requiring the tibialis anterior to work harder decelerating the forefoot to the ground.

O   **Which types of sports/activities are most likely to produce lateral shin splints involving the Peroneal musculature?**

Sports/activities requiring lateral mobility, multidirectional and/or eversional type motion.

O   **What are some typical radiographic findings seen in tibial stress fracture?**

Periosteal reaction, cortical hypertrophy, endosteal canal narrowing due to endosteal reaction, possible lucent fracture line. Early radiographs may be negative and may require Tc99 bone scan (hot spot) or MRI (dec. signal intensity of endosteal canal on T1 and increased signal intensity of endosteal canal on T2 and/or STIR).

O   **What is the most common location of Tibial Stress fractures in runners?**

Middle to lower 1/3 of the Tibia along the posterior medial tibial ridge.

O   **What is the most common location of Fibular stress fractures?**

Most occur in the distal ¼ of the fibula, in adults about 4-6 cm. Superior to the medial malleolus.

❍   **What are the pathomechanics behind the development of "Chronic Compartment Syndrome" of the leg?**

A higher than normal, increased resting compartment pressure due to a tight fascial bag around a particular muscle or group of muscles. With exercise, blood flow to the muscular compartment increases, increasing volume of an already tight compartment resulting in a pathologic elevation of intercompartmental pressure resulting in ischemic type symptoms. While this is not a surgical emergency (differing from acute compartment syndrome), elective fasciotomy may reduce or eliminate the problem.

❍   **What is "Tennis Leg?"**

An acute posterior calf strain, usually the medial head of the Gastrocnemius or possibly the Soleus. Previously thought to be a rupture of the Plantaris tendon.

❍   **What is the usual mechanism resulting in "Tennis Leg?"**

Usually occurs in a fatigued/fatiguing Gastroc/Soleus. The muscle is eccentrically loaded/stretched as body weight moves forward over the foot/leg. This is followed by a forceful, sudden contraction of the Gastroc/Soleus resulting in strain of the involved muscle.

❍   **What is the "Q Angle?"**

This is the quadriceps angle or relationship of the line of pull of the quads to the line of pull of the patellar tendon. It is formed by a line connecting the ASIS to the midpoint/center of the patellar intersecting with a line from the midpoint/center of the patella to the tibial tubercle. The normal angle is between 10-18 degrees and is abnormal if either too high or too low.

❍   **Pathologically, what does the Q Angle reflect?**

Tracking of the Patella in the intercondylar notch of the Femur. An abnormal Q angle suggests the possibility of abnormal Patellar tracking and a possible mechanical cause for Patellofemoral Pain Syndrome.

❍   **What is the "common denominator" in Patellofemoral Pain Syndrome?**

Abnormal, increased Patellofemoral contact pressures.

❍   **When the Patella subluxes or dislocates, which direction does this usually occur?**

Laterally.

❍   **When evaluating muscle activity and strength in chronic Patellar subluxation and Patellofemoral Pain Syndrome, which muscle frequently appears weak and atrophic?**

The Vastus Medialis Obliquis (Part of the Quads).

❍   **In evaluating a knee, what is the "Panic" or "Apprehension Sign?"**

When attempting to sublux the Patella laterally to evaluate the mobility of the Patella, the patient will respond with panic or apprehension and may respond by withdrawing, contracting the quads, etc. to avoid the discomfort previously experienced with Patellar subluxation or laxity.

❍   **What is "Clark's Test" and when is it used?**

This is a test to evaluate the status (inflammation/irregularity, etc) of the retropatellar surface as a cause of retropatellar pain in Patellofemoral Pain Syndrome and Chondromalacia. The Patella is distracted and held distally following which the quads are contracted. The Patella is thereby forced against the femoral condyles which may produce pain and crepitation associated with retropatellar surface inflammation, irregularity, etc. The exam should be performed with the knee mildly flexed as compared to fully extended to avoid trapping redundant synovium between the Patella and Femur which would also produce pain and a false positive finding.

○ **In Plica Syndrome of the knee, symptoms generally occur in which area of the knee?**

Peripatellarly, usually over the medial/superior-medial area of the adjacent femoral condyle.

○ **What are some of the typical pathomechanics which may result in Plica Syndrome of the knee?**

Direct blow to the knee.
High intensity flexion/extension activities.
Excessive/abnormal pronation stretching the plica due to tibial rotation and valgus stress at the knee.

In any case, the plica, a band of redundant tissue which usually resorbs following birth, but in this case remains, becomes thickened, fibrotic and inelastic due to inflammation and hence resulting in pain.

○ **List the differential diagnoses in patients with suspected Patellofemoral Pain Syndrome.**

Chondromalacia Patellae; Plica Syndrome.
Meniscal injury.
Chronic Patellar Subluxation.
Synovitis.
Fat Pad Entrapment Syndrome (infrapatellar fat pad) = Hoffa's Syndrome.
Bursitis.

○ **List the possible mechanical etiologies resulting in Patellar tendonitis in athletes.**

Excessive jumping activities.
Tight hamstrings (quads have to work harder to extend knee).
Tight quads (tendon becomes stretched with activities involving excessive knee flexion).
Excessive midstance knee flexion, i.e., long leg compensation.
Under striding.

○ **What is Osgood-Schlatter's Disease?**

Traction apophysitis of the tibial tubercle due to excessive tension of the Patellar tendon. Occurs most commonly between 10-15 years of age in young athletes involved in jumping sports or activities requiring increased tension on the Patellar tendon.

○ **Pes Anserine tendonitis involves inflammation of which muscular insertions?**

Sartorius; Gracilis; Semitendinosus.

○ **What is the usual mechanism behind the development of IT (iliotibial) Band Syndrome?**

With knee flexion and extension, the IT band snaps or rubs back and forth over the lateral femoral condyle. The repetitive "friction" results in inflammation and pain and, hence, the name ITB "Friction" Syndrome.

○ **What might be some mechanical etiologies of ITB Syndrome?**

Tight IT band; Cavus foot (shock dissipation in ITB); Excessive ITB stress/fatigue (hills/sloped or crested roads); Varus deformities (genu varum, tibial varum, rearfoot varus, compensation for short limb, etc.); Excessive internal tibial rotation which tightens ITB, (ie. Excessive pronation, long limb compensation.)

○   What test evaluates the tightness of the IT Band?

The "Ober" test. Lying on the opposite side of the leg being tested, the medial side of the knee being tested should be able to reach the table with minimal to no resistance. Restriction of the medial side from reaching the exam table may be due to tightness of the IT Band on the lateral side of the limb.

○   What are the usual mechanical causes of Popliteus Muscle Syndrome seen in a runner?

Excessive downhill running, displacing the femur anteriorly on the tibia stressing the Popliteus which limits anterior displacement of the femur on the tibia; Factors which result in excessive external tibial rotation; Factors which result in excessive internal femoral rotation (the Popliteus internally rotates the tibia and prevents anterior displacement of the Femur on the Tibia. Therefore, anything that excessively externally rotates the Tibia, excessively internally rotates the Femur or produces excessive anterior displacement stress of the Femur may stress the Popliteus).

○   The discomfort in Popliteus Muscle Syndrome would occur in which area of the knee?

Posterolateral.

○   Most chronic problems involving the Achilles tendon occur within 2-6 cm superior to the Calcaneal insertion. Why does this frequently occur in this area?

This is an area of reduced vascularity or the so called "watershed" area which makes this area vulnerable to injury and with a reduced healing potential.

○   What is the relationship of excessive, abnormal pronation to chronic Achilles tendonitis?

Due to:
- Bowstringing of the Achilles tendon as the foot pronates, tightening the medial side of the tendon.
- Torque or "wringing" effect of the tendon. The tibia remains internally rotated in the pronated foot while the knee is extending in midstance and propulsion producing a conflicting torque force on the tendon. The wringing effect may also cause tendon "blanching" and cyclic periods of further reduced vascularity.
- In the foot with compensatory pronation due to equinus, the Achilles tendon is tight (reduced flexibility) increasing the tension within the tendon.

○   What is the usual appearance of the runner with chronic Achilles tendonitis?

Most often male (approximately 80%), average age around 40.

○   How does foot strike contribute to the development of chronic Achilles tendonitis?

In rearfoot strikers, there is a higher vibration resonance within the tendon which is also under higher eccentric tension at heel strike. In midfoot strikers, there is a resulting increased eccentric muscle decelerator activity as the heel is eccentrically lowered to the ground following heel strike. Both situations may increase tension within the Achilles tendon.

○   What is the "Thompson Test?"

This is a manual test used to evaluate the integrity of the Achilles tendon. The calf is squeezed (Gastroc/Soleus only, avoiding squeezing of the deep posterior muscle group). Plantarflexion of the foot suggest at least a partially intact Achilles tendon. Absence of plantarflexion of the foot suggests discontinuity of the Achilles tendon.

❍ **What are some manual tests used to evaluate the integrity of the ligamentous structures of the ankle following acute ankle injury?**

Anterior drawer (pull test) to evaluate the Anterior Talofibular ligament. Calcaneal inversion (Talar Tilt) to evaluate the Calcaneofibular ligament when it is positioned parallel to the long axis of the leg. Eversion stress test to evaluate the integrity of the Superficial Deltoid. External rotation test to evaluate the integrity of the Deep Deltoid fibers. Dorsiflexion and external rotation to evaluate the Tibiofibular ligaments.

❍ **To what does the Salter-Harris classification refer?**

The epiphyseal plate in children.

❍ **What is the weakest zone in the epiphyseal plate, or plane of cleavage in most epiphyseal plate fractures in children?**

The Zone of Provisional Calcification

❍ **Describe the 5 main forms of epiphyseal plate fractures.**

S-H I: Fracture only through the plate without epiphyseal or metaphyseal involvement.
S-H II: Fracture along the plate with a projection out through the metaphysis producing a metaphyseal spike ("Thurston-Holland Sign").
S-H III: Fracture through the joint surface, longitudinally through the epiphysis to the plate and then transversely out through the epiphyseal plate.
S-H IV: Fracture through the joint surface, longitudinally through the epiphysis, across the plate and terminating out through the metaphysis.
S-H V: Compression injury of the epiphyseal plate, partial or complete.

❍ **The classical description of a Jones fracture of the 5th metatarsal is:**

A transversely oriented fracture line distal to the styloid process of the 5th metatarsal in the proximal portion of the bone.

❍ **In Subluxed Cuboid Syndrome, there may be an associated tendonitis of which tendon?**

The Peroneus Longus.

❍ **Describe the mechanical etiologies of extensor tendonitis as may be seen in the athlete.**

Weak Tibialis Anterior with extensor substitution; compression from underlying bony prominence; excessive dorsiflexion activities (extensor assist); "step on" injury of the forefoot/midfoot.

❍ **In a "saddle bone" deformity in an athlete (1st met-medial cuneiform dorsal exostosis), clinical symptoms and complaints are most frequently the result of what?**

Compression of soft tissue structures (tendon, nerve, etc.) between the dorsal exostosis and the extrinsic pressure from the shoe, resulting in the development of symptoms.

❍ **What is the usual mechanism behind the development of retrocalcaneal bursitis in the athlete?**

Pressure between the posterior-superior bursal surface of the calcaneus and the Achilles tendon with resulting inflammation of the bursa with swelling and pain. This may be due to an enlargement of the posterior surface of the calcaneus (Haglund's deformity), an abnormal position of the calcaneus (high Calcaneal Inclination angle with the bursal surface pushed against the Achilles tendon), extrinsic pressure from the counter of the shoe over the area of the bursal surface, and possibly rotational motion of the calcaneus with frictional pressure created in the area of the retrocalcaneal bursa. This is besides other systemic causes such as sero-negative and sero-positive arthropathies which are only incidental to the athlete.

GENERAL CONCEPTS

○ **What are some characteristic changes in gait between the walking and running gait?**

Changes in running gait
- Narrowing of base of gait
- Decreasing angle of gait
- Lowered center of gravity
- Increased varus position of the heel at heel contact
- Increase proportion of airborn (swing) time to stance (ground contact) time
- Changes in landing (contact) patterns as speed increases (i.e., land on forefoot/forefoot strike and rock back to heel)
- Increased proportion of time in propulsion (forefoot contact time) vs. time spent on rearfoot.
- Increase in ground reactive forces (Newton's 2nd Law - Force mass x acceleration)
- Increased importance of swing phase to maintain momentum
- Change in stride length

○ **How can a runner increase their speed?**

Increase the cadence (strides per minute) or increase the stride length.

○ **What constitutes the beginning of "push off" or "follow through" phase?**

Toe off occurs.

○ **How would tight hip flexors reduce "push off" efficiency?**

Tight hip flexors would limit hip extension/hyperextension, which would decrease the push off angle, thereby reducing push off efficiency and speed.

○ **Describe 2 factors which would decreased the effectiveness of the "float" or "double float" phase in runners.**

Weak hamstrings/hip extensors with decreased retrograde force against the ground, thereby reducing float.
Weak plantarflexors which would decrease the push off force.
Weak quads/hip flexors which would decrease the force of the leg moving forward in the air, reducing momentum.

○ **What are the major problems experienced with over striding? With under striding?**

In over striding, there tends to be increased shock absorption related problems as well as forced knee hyperextension. In under striding, there tends to be excessive sagittal plane stress with anterior ankle impingement problems, increased stress on the Achilles tendon and excessive patellar tendon stress (eccentric) with knee flexion and increased patellofemoral pressures.

○ **What is the purpose of knee flexion which occurs just after "foot strike?"**

The knee flexes not just as a more proximal shock absorber but the knee flexion allows "unlocking" of the knee which allows the tibia to internally rotation to allow talar adduction and subtalar joint pronation.

○ **How does the "take off" phase in runners contribute to the development of forefoot problems?**

During "take off," there is the second peak in ground reactive force where force is concentrated on the forefoot. In the faster runner or sprinter, the majority of ground contact time is on the forefoot with an elongated "take off" phase which maximizes forces on the forefoot.

❍   What are the different ways to classify limb length discrepancies?

Structural – 1 limb is structurally/anatomically longer than the other.
Functional – both limbs are of equal length but one leg functions shorter or longer than the other, i.e. STJ pronation shortening a leg.
Combined – elements of both structural and functional.
Environmental – both limbs are of equal length but the athlete may function asymmetrically as a result of the environment or surface they are running on, such as the side of a crested road, side of a hill, etc.

❍   **What are some typical limb compensations occurring in a structurally long limb?**

MTJ pronation; STJ pronation; Excessive midstance knee flexion; Excessive hip flexion and/or internal rotation

❍   **How does the back compensate for a limb length discrepancy?**

In a simple, single curve, the back compensates with a functional scoliosis with the back concave to the long side and convex to the short side which results in a shoulder drop on the long side. With a more complex curve, the back may attempt to stabilize the curve, resulting in 2 curves with the lumbar region concave to the long and thoracic convex to the long and conversely on the short. In this second scenario, the shoulder drop may level out or become lower on the short.

❍   **The best physical indicator of the short or long side in either a functional or structural limb length discrepancy is:**

The level of the iliac crest which would be higher on the long and lower on the short (not considering compensations for a structural limb length discrepancy)

❍   **Where do most limb compensations occur in structural limb length discrepancies?**

Most occur on the long side since most compensations which occur on the long side tend to be "passive" requiring less initial energy expenditure, i.e. STJ pronation. The compensations have a tendency to occur in the direction of least initial energy expenditure but only if ample motion is available in the compensating joint.

❍   **In limb length discrepancies, which side tends to be more symptomatic and why?**

Most symptoms occur on the long side since most compensations occur on the long side. Also the stance phase tends to be longer on the long side and the long side, because of the two previous factors, result in increased stresses and loads to the long side.

❍   **Describe different methods for determining or evaluating a limb length discrepancy.**

True Limb length – ASIS to malleolus (doesn't take into consideration anything distal to the ankle).
Apparent limb length – umbilicus to the malleolus (very unreliable due to positions of the umbilicus).
Standing limb lengths – considers the length of the limb from pelvis to the floor and therefore, more appropriate. This should be done in angle and base of gait and in neutral and relaxed calcaneal stance to help determine structural vs. functional and associated compensations (fully, partially, uncompensated).

Trial lifts – add lifts until pelvis is level.
Segmental lengths – floor to malleolus, malleolus to knee joint line, knee, joint line to ASIS, etc.
Sitting – one knee higher than other.

Lying with knees flexed – one knee higher than the other.

○   **What are some findings which may be observed on gait analysis in patients with a limb length discrepancy?**

The head may be tilted/tipped towards either the long or short side. The shoulders may be level but may be dropped on either the long or the short side. The arm swing may be asymmetrical, increased or decreased on either the long or short side. The back presents with a functional scoliotic curve. There may be asymmetrical transverse plane motion of the hip increased or decreased on either the long or short side. The pelvis may be dropped, generally to the short side and elevated on the long. The knee may demonstrate increased flexion on the long side in midstance or, in some cases a genu recurvatum. Unilateral pronation on the long side with abducted and widened gait on the long side or unilateral supination, early heel off on the short side.

○   **What would be the difference in treatment philosophies between a functional vs. structural limb length discrepancy?**

In a functional discrepancy, identify the functional etiology, (ie, intrinsic foot biomechanical abnormality, equinus, muscle imbalance, etc.) and treat the etiology directly. In a structural discrepancy, a lift is added to the short side, beginning with a lift generally ¼ to ¼ the amount of the measured difference and add lift incrementally to the short side only as needed to reduce symptoms.

○   **What are various parts of the running/athletic shoe uppers?**

Heel counter, heel collar (pull tab/notch), toe box, tongue, eyeletsi, vamp, shank.

○   **What factors will increase the effectiveness of the heel counter of the running shoe?**

Firm counter (plastic or more rigid material); Reinforced counter (ie increased foxing, multiple materials); Higher counter; Longer counter; Counter firmly attached to the midsole; Counter-midsole junction reinforced by a heel stabilizer; Counter on a firm midsole.

○   **What are typical midsole materials and how are they measured?**

Most common materials for a midsole are EVA (Ethyl Vinyl Acetate) and Polyurethane. EVA tends to provide a more cushioned feel and tend to be less durable and "bottom out" faster. Polyurethane tends to be more durable but with generally a less cushioned feel. The midsole is often measured in density in durometers with a low durometer (softer) material about 25 and a denser, firmer durometer around 45+.

○   **What is the difference between a board/conventional/machine/cement lasted shoe vs. a slip/moccasin lasted shoe?**

In a board/etc. lasted shoe, the uppers are glued/stitched to the periphery of the midsole with the center of the upper open plantarly to the midsole. This opening is covered by a cardboard/fiberboard plate. This board last tends to make the shoe stiffer with more torsional stability. In a slip lasted shoe, the uppers cover the entire plantar surface, stitched together plantarly and the material is attached to the midsole with the foot covered on the sides and plantarly entirely by the uppers. The slip lasted shoe tends to be more flexible with a snugger/improved fit.

○   **What is a combination lasted shoe?**

The typical combination lasted shoe is board lasted in the rearfoot and slip lasted in the forefoot to provide rearfoot stability and forefoot flexibility and fit.

○   **How is the shape of the shoe influenced by the foot?**

Shoes can be described as straight, slightly curved, semi-curved and curved lasted. Generally, the shape of the foot should be matched by the shape of the shoe. If the runner has a rectus foot, choose a straight lasted shoe. If the runner has an adductus foot, a curved last may be more appropriate. Therefore, the shape of the shoe should compare to the shape of the foot to avoid excessive medial or lateral crowding. In a pronated foot, try to select as straight a shoe as possible which provides more medial support and stability which may be beneficial with excessive pronation.

○   **What are some common ways to increase the shock absorbing capabilities of a running shoe?**

Use a lower durometer (lower density) midsole.
Perforated midsoles (transverse perforations).
Various midsole modifications:
- air or gas bags, entrapped air in chambers
- silicone or shock absorbing gels or liquids
- compressible, flexible platforms (hytrel strings/trampolines)
- compressible/flexible vertical walls or pillars).

○   **What is the "sock liner" and what is its purpose?**

The sock liner is the insole and should provide a smooth, internal conformed liner, assist in reducing shock and increasing cushion, reduce shear and friction and absorb sweat.

○   **How would one go about evaluating a shoe wear pattern?**

Wear patterns may reflect abnormal function or shoe/foot compatibility.
- Look at the uppers to see if they are bulging over the medial or lateral sides of the shoes which would reflect fit. Also look for areas of wear through, ie toe box, etc., which may reflect areas of pressure or crowding.
- Look at the counter to see if it is vertical or tipped medially or laterally, if the counter is firm or cracked and if there is evidence of wear in the inside of the counter. All would reflect the amount of rearfoot motion in the shoe or the position of the heel during gait.
- Look at the insole/sock liner to see if there is excessive wear reflecting areas of increased pressure or friction. Also see if the foot impression is symmetrical on the insole which would reflect adequate fit rather than crowded to one side or the other which would reflect abnormal or improper fit.
- Look at the midsole to determine if there are areas of wear or compression which may reflect abnormal biomechanics, ie., medial compression in an uncontrolled, excessively pronated foot and lateral compression in an uncontrolled supinated foot or with increased varus of the rearfoot. Also evaluate the midsole for any modifications, ie., shock absorption devices and their appropriateness.
- Look at the outsole for areas of excessive wear which may reflect abnormal biomechanical function depending on the location of the abnormal wear, such as in the toe box in uncompensated/partially compensated equinus, medial in the rearfoot in the excessively pronated or valgus foot or excessive lateral wear in the supinated or varus foot.
- Is the wear pattern symmetrical, unilateral or paradoxical which may reflect an asymmetry problem.
- Is there any torque in the shoe which may reflect frontal plane abnormalities or compensations.

○   **What effect does a lateral midsole flare have on athletic shoe function?**

The flare may provide some support against inversion as it hits the ground at the most lateral aspect of the midsole and rapidly everts the foot. However, this may aggravate pronatory problems because of this rapid eversion, ie., posterior tibial tendonitis or posterior shin splints.

○   **What is a biased heel and what effect does it have on a running shoe?**

A biased heel or "shin splint cut off" is a rounded wedged off area of the midsole in the posterior heel region. This allows a slower and more gradual transition from heel contact to foot flat, thereby reducing anterior muscular stress and strain, resulting in improvement of Tibialis Anterior or Extensor muscle overuse. However, in runners with Achilles tendon problems, heel contact may be more posterior than normal with increased stress on the Achilles which may aggravate an Achilles tendon problem.

○   **What is the difference between a concentric and eccentric muscle contraction?**

In a concentric contraction, the muscle is contracting and shortening. In an eccentric contraction, the muscle is contracting but lengthening (also called "negative" contractions)

○   **What is the difference between isometric, isotonic and isokinetic exercise?**

In isometric exercise, muscle is contraction but against a fixed resistance, thereby producing no motion. This tends to strengthen only this segment of the range of motion.

In isotonic exercise, a weight is moved through a range of motion. The weight may be affected by gravity if lifted or lowered vertically. Not all points in a range of motion are of equal strength and, therefore, the maximal weight which can be moved through a full range of motion is only that which can be accommodated at the weakest segment of the arc of motion.

In isokinetic exercise, the resistance is time controlled. No actual weight is used but a bar or device which is allowed to travel only at a set maximal speed is moved through a range of motion. If maximal effort is exerted, maximal resistance is obtained by restriction of the bar motion. If lesser effort is applied, the bar may still move at the same speed but with less resistance and, therefore, less benefit.

○   **What is delayed onset muscle soreness (D.O.M.S.)?**

This is a transient muscle condition with soreness and tightness which most frequently occurs following resumption of an exercise program or following particularly intense activity, believed to be due to mild tearing/damage to connective tissue surrounding muscle fiber, bundle and muscle. The condition is self-limiting and may be relieved by passive stretch. This is the "day after soreness" which we have all experienced at some time.

○   **How does delayed onset muscle soreness differ from exertional rhabdomyolysis?**

Delayed onset muscle soreness is a self-limiting, non-critical condition. Rhabdomyolysis is a condition of extreme muscular exertion with actual muscle fiber disruption and cellular death where muscle contents are eventually spilled into the serum, filtered in the kidney and excreted in the urine. Rhabdomyolysis is potentially more severe with disruptions of serum potassium, phosphate, uric acid and their consequences as well as renal complications from the breakdown of myoglobin which in some conditions may be nephrotoxic and compartmental edema due to inflammation as the result of muscle cell breakdown.

○   **What serum abnormalities may be seen with Rhabdomyolysis?**

With the loss of muscle cell contents, muscle enzymes may be elevated in the serum, such as aldolase and CPK. Also elevated may be SGOT and LDH, succinic dehydrogenase, creatine and potassium and phosphorus/phosphate. The presence of myoglobin in the serum doesn't stain the serum red as would hemoglobin in hemolytic anemias. (Urine with myoglobin however will test positive for occult blood by Hematest but will not show RBC's or RBC fragments microscopically).

○   **What is a muscle strain?**

A strain is a stretch or tear of a muscle which may be acute due to a sudden violent event (muscle contraction or violent stretch) or may be chronic due to an overuse, microtraumatic etiology where due to repetitive contractions, the muscle may eventually strain.

○   **In general, which types of muscles are more prone to muscle strain?**

More powerful muscles are more prone to strain because of their inherent activity and requirements. More phasic muscles are more prone to strain due to the repetitive nature of their contractions. Muscles subject to more ballistic and faster activities are more prone to strain because of their being subject to more violent contractions. Also, muscles which are inflexible or weak, creating muscle ratio imbalances are also more prone to strain.

○   **What is a muscle cramp and how is it treated?**

A muscle cramp is a painful muscular contraction generally beginning as an area of increased electrical activity in the muscle, producing initially a single focus of fasciculation and then spreading erratically throughout the muscle. This generally occurs following prolonged activity or muscular work and may be fatigue related resulting in the inability of the muscle to adequately relax or creating a state of hyperexcitability where the muscle is more easily stimulated. Other factors such as fluid and electrolyte depletion (ie. potassium, sodium, calcium, magnesium) with dehydration, sweating and diuresis may contribute to the problem. The initial cramp is generally treated by slow, passive stretching. Water and electrolyte imbalances and deficiencies should also be corrected.

○   **When using an MRI to evaluate a athletic injury what is a T1 weighted image? T2 weighted image? STIR? TE? TR?**

A T1 weighted image or a "fat weighted" image, has a short TE and short TR and fat has a high signal intensity (bright) as a reference. Good for anatomical appearance. Tissues with a short T1 relaxation time appear bright on T1 weighted images, ie. fat.

A T2 weighted image or "water weighted" image has a long TE and long TR and water has a high signal intensity (bright) as a reference. Good for identifying areas of fluid collection/inflammatory edema, etc. Tissues with short T2 relaxation times appear bright with increased signal intensity on T2 weighted images, ie. water.

A STIR is a "fat suppression" image where fat appears dark, thereby emphasizing fluid collections even more emphatically than a T2 weighted image. The TE and TR can be either like T1 or T2 but most often like T1.

TE is the time to echo or receive emitted energy. This is short in T1 images and long in T2 images. The nuclei are "excited" by an external energy source and eventually release this "excited energy" and sampled at the echo time.

TR is the time to repeat the external energy stimulation/source (radiofrequency energy) to excite atomic nuclei.

○   **What would Achilles tendonitis look like on MRI?**

The tendon should be normally uniformly black without any intratendinous increased signals and should be of even size without any particular areas of enlargement. In Achilles tendonitis, findings may range from widening or thickening of the tendon without change in signal intensity to areas of intermediate signal (streaks/"clouds") within the tendon on T1 weighted images and areas of high signal intensity with inflammatory edema on T2 or STIR images. There may also be decreased signal intensity in posterior triangle fat on T1 due to inflammatory changes in the triangle.

○   **How would tenosynovitis appear on MRI in an athlete suspected of having tenosynovitis?**

Due to increased fluid in the tendon sheath, there would be in intermediate signal around the tendon on T1 and an increased, high intensity signal around the tendon on T2 and STIR.

○   **How would bone contusion appear on MRI?**

There would be in ill-defined area of decreased signal on T1 within the cancellous area of the bone with an increased signal intensity due to fluid in the same area on T2 and STIR. This ill-defined area generally appears reticulated.

○   **How would stress fracture appear on MRI?**

There may be a focus of decreased signal intensity in the area of the stress fracture on T1 in the medullary/cancellous region with increased signal intensity on T2 and STIR in the area due to medullary edema and hemorrhage. There may be evident an area of cortical irregularity and periosteal reaction would be identified by a low signal intensity linear line which would parallel the bone with an intervening area of increased signal intensity immediately adjacent to the cortex.

○   **What is Wolff's Law?**

Wolff's Law states that "every change in form and/or function of bone is followed by certain definite changes in the internal architecture and secondary alterations to the external configuration" of bone. Bone will respond to stress by altering it external and internal architecture/configuration. When repetitive stress exceeds the ability of bone to remodel, stress fracture may occur.

○   **What is the piezoelectric effect in bone and how does it affect bone remodeling?**

Since bone is largely crystalline in nature, as bone bends, an electric current is induced in bone by the piezoelectric effect (the bending of crystals inducing an electrical current). The tendon side of the bone becomes relatively electropositive and the compression side, relatively electronegative. Current flow is from positive to negative. This current induction stimulates bone remodeling.

○   **What stress is the usual cause for long bone failure in stress fracture?**

Bending of the bone because of abnormal muscle pull or other mechanical etiology producing tension stress.

○   **When a stress fracture occurs by compression, how does this usually differ in radiographic appearance from a typical tension failure? Where is this most common in the lower extremity?**

Bones with stress failure due to compression most frequently have a more sclerotic appearance with trabecular disruption. This is typical in the calcaneus, possibly the navicular and proximal femur.

○   **How would you best define "stress fracture?"**

A focal, structural weakness or defect during bone remodeling in response to repeated applications of subthreshold stress.

○   **How does muscle contraction and muscle fatigue result in stress fracture?**

Repetitive muscle contraction exerts cyclic bending stress on bone, which may stimulate remodeling. Muscle normally assists in absorbing shock. When muscle becomes fatigued by repeated activity, more shock needs to be dissipated by bone at focal bending points resulting in eventual bone failure.

○   **What is the Kroening and Shelton Classification of stress fracture?**

This is a classification system based upon radiographic appearance of the stress fracture.
  • Linear – generally in long bones with a fine radiolucent cleft appearance with a possible "knife slice" fracture defect. Generally heals with abundant callus.

- Periosteal – also generally in long bones but without a fracture line being evident. Also heals with marked callus.
- Sclerotic – generally seen in bones with large cancellous concentration, usually as a result of compressive forces. The fracture appears as an internal cancellous sclerosis without any apparent cortical defect or periosteal reaction.
- Fragmentary – most frequently in the metatarsals where multiple fracture fragments are visualized with a comminuted appearance
- Combined/mixed – elements of multiples of the above

O   **What is the general initial treatment of acute, macrotraumatic injuries occurring to athletes?**

PRICE therapy
- P = protect
- R = rest (the area of injury)
- I = ice
- C = Compression
- E = elevation

TENDONS

❍ **What is the difference between a tendon transfer versus a tendon transposition?**

In a tendon transfer procedure, the tendon is detached at its insertion and relocated to a new attachment, whereas, a transposition involves rerouting the course of a tendon without detachment.

❍ **Describe a tendon's blood supply.**

Three main sources are responsible for providing nourishment to the tendon.
1. Muscular branches at the myotendinous junction.
2. Vessels at the tendo-osseous junction (periosteum and bone).
3. Blood vessels running in the mesotenon or paratenon. (Tendons also receive nutrition from lymphatic and synovial fluid.)

❍ **Of the sources of blood supply to a tendon, which supplies the majority of the blood?**

Paratenon and mesotenon.

❍ **What are the stages in tendon healing for a surgically repaired tendon?**

Inflammatory (exudative) phase seen initially in 48-72 hours.
Fibroblastic (formative) phase at beginning approximately at day 5 in which collagen is laid down in random fashion.
Remodeling (organizational) phase from 15 to 28 days in which collagen is laid parallel to the tendon.

❍ **Which muscles of the lower leg are predominantly swing phase muscles?**

Tibialis anterior, extensor hallucis longus, extensor digitorum longus, and peroneus tertius.

❍ **After primary repair of a tendon, when should the patient begin isometric exercises?**

3 weeks.

❍ **What is the watershed area of a tendon?**

Area of low vascularity of the tendon, which can be a common area of rupture.

❍ **How does the anatomical arrangement of blood supply to the tendon contribute to weakened areas?**

Of the sources described, the musculotendinous and tendo-osseous vessels supply the proximal and distal 1/3 of the tendon. The paratenon or mesotenon supply the middle 1/3. Between these regions are areas of decreased vascularity resulting in weakened portions of the tendon.

❍ **Which of the tendons that cross the ankle joint lack a synovial tendon sheath?**

Achilles tendon and plantaris.

❍ **Of the tendons that have a synovial tendon sheath in the foot and ankle, which sheath extends the most distal?**

Extensor hallucis longus synovial tendon sheath.

O   **Name and describe the supporting tissue of a tendon that has a direct course from its origin to insertion.**

Paratenon – loose elastic areolar tissue that move with the tendon during contraction.

O   **Describe the course of a tendon with a synovial tendon sheath.**

A tendon that is subject to pressure such as one coursing beneath retinacula or one that changes direction or rounds a corner through a fibro-osseous tunnel.

O   **Which tendons of the foot and ankle share a common synovial tendon sheath?**

1. Peroneus longus and peroneus brevis and 2. extensor digitorum longus and peroneus tertius.

O   **What kind of deformity must be present for a tendon transfer to be effective?**

Flexible deformity in which there is a dynamic muscular imbalance.

O   **What is the name of the most basic molecule of a tendon?**

Tropocollagen.

O   **Describe the transition of cells at the insertion of a tendon into bone.**

Collagen fibers to fibrocartilage, which become calcified and organized into bone.

O   **What are these transitional fibers at the insertion of a tendon into bone known as?**

Perforating fibers of Sharpey or Sharpey's fibers.

O   **What structure of the tendon has been shown to be the most proliferative structure in the tendon repair process?**

Epitenon.

O   **Describe the strength of a healing tendon during the first week status post primary repair.**

The strength of healing tendon at this time is no greater than the suture (usually until 10-14 days).

O   **What is a tendon callus? When does it form?**

The tendon callus (also known as fibroblastic splint) forms during the first week of tendon healing. It is a bridge of serous and granulation tissue (from the inflammatory cell exudates) that forms within the peri-sheath tissue or gap zone.

O   **What acts as a fulcrum for the peroneus longus tendon?**

Cuboid.

O   **Can a muscle/tendon be "retrained" if transferred out of phase?**

Yes – post-op rehab is imperative.

O   **What tendon transfer procedure would be indicated for a rigidly plantarflexed first metatarsal?**

None – deformity must be flexible for tendon transfer to be indicated unless rigid deformity is fixed prior to tendon procedure.

O   **When performing manual muscle testing, at what position must the muscle be placed?**

At its end range of motion.

O   **If a patient can move only against gravity alone without resistance, what grade of strength would this be?**

Three, fair.

O   **Does a tendon transfer or lengthening procedure effect the strength of the tendon involved? Explain.**

Yes – usually it is equal to a loss of 1 grade of muscle strength on manual muscle examination .

O   **What (if any) is the effect of prolonged immobilization in the tendon repair process?**

Retarded tensile strength of union as well as increase chance of adhesions.

O   **What tendon transfer procedure is indicated for spasticity of the triceps surae?**

Murphy procedure – anterior advancement of the Achilles tendon.

O   **What tendon transfer could be useful in the correction of a hallux varus deformity?**

Abductor hallucis transferred from the medial to lateral side of the hallux (adjunctive procedure).

O   **A patient presents with a reducible hammertoe deformity of the hallux. What tendon procedure could be indicated?**

Jones tendon transfer.

O   **What other procedure would be performed with the above tendon transfer and why?**

IPJ fusion – this is performed to prevent hammering at the IPJ after transfer.

O   **What structures must be preserved at all costs for a tendon to heal properly?**

Peritendinous structures (paratenon, mesotenon…).

O   **Following tendon repair, when should the patient be allowed to have a gradual return to activity?**

4 weeks.

O   **Why is early movement essential after a tendon transfer is performed?**

To prevent long lasting adhesion formation.

O   **Where is the watershed area of the Achilles tendon?**

2-6 cm proximal to the calcaneal insertion.

O   **What is the grace period for primary repair of a tendon laceration?**

6-8 hours.

O   **Describe the innervation of tendons.**

Three types of nerve endings innervate tendons. Paciniform which receives touch, golgi tendon organs which perceive stretch, and free nerve endings which transmit pain sensation.

O   **After performing the Hibbs procedure, what (if anything) is done with the distal stumps of the transferred tendons and why?**

Distal stumps of the longus tendons are sutured into the corresponding brevis tendons to allow for active dorsiflexion of the toes.

O   **Describe the rerouting of the tendon in the Jones suspension procedure.**

The EHL is transected at the IPJ of the hallux and rerouted through a medial to lateral drill hole in the head of the first metatarsal and sutured back onto itself dorsally. The distal stump of the tendon is attached to the EHB to maintain some extensor function of the hallux.

O   **A patient with a dropfoot deformity undergoes a tibialis posterior tendon transfer. Describe the phasic activity involved pre and post transfer.**

Stance phase preop to swing phase postop.

O   **Through what structure must the tibialis posterior tendon be passed in the above procedure.**

Interosseous membrane of the leg.

O   **Where is the tenodesis site for the Hibbs procedure?**

Base of third metatarsal or lateral cuneiform.

O   **Where is the watershed region of the tibialis posterior tendon?**

Behind the medial malleolus.

O   **What are the four types of posterior tibial tendon rupture?**

Group 1 is avulsion of the tendon usually 1-2 cm proximal to its navicular insertion. Group 2 is a midsubstance tear around the medial malleolus, Group 3 is in-continuity longitudinal tear without complete rupture, and Group 4 is tenosynovitis without visible disruption.

O   **Which tendon lies adjacent to bone in the fibular groove.**

Peroneus brevis.

O   **When the Achilles tendon is ruptured, which fibers are most usually ruptured first?**

Posterior fibers.

○ **Describe the Thompson-Doherty test.**

Used to test the integrity of the Achilles tendon. (Good for testing total rupture) The patient is prone with his/her foot hanging off the table. The calf is squeezed and the foot is watched for its response. Absence of plantarflexion is a positive test and indicates severe rupture of the tendon. If plantarflexion occurs, this is a negative test and indicates integrity of the tendon.

○ **Would you expect a patient with a total rupture of the Achilles tendon to perform active plantarflexion? Explain.**

Yes – utilizing the posterior and lateral muscle groups.

○ **What is the strongest part of the musculotendinous unit?**

Tendon.

○ **List some predisposing factors to rupture of a tendon.**

Cortisone injections, calcification of tendon, tenosynovitis, tendonitis, arthritis, infection, underlying medical conditions, age, decreased blood supply to tendon, biomechanical abnormalities, and other disease processes of the tendon.

○ **A patient presents with a dorsal medial laceration of the foot. Describe your clinical examination to rule out an EHL tendon laceration.**

Have patient do active dorsiflexion at the IPJ against resistance. If a dysfunction is present, IPJ joint extension should be lacking. MTPJ dorsiflexion would still occur because of the functioning EHB.

○ **What is the most common cause of tendon rupture of the posterior tibialis tendon?**

Chronic or acute stress on an already degenerated tendon.

○ **Can an X-ray contribute to the diagnosis of an Achilles tendon rupture? Explain.**

Yes, by examining Kager's triangle, which can be blunted superiorly because of retraction of the proximal stump. Also, the appearance of the triangle may be changed as compared to the contralateral side secondary to swelling and hematoma.

○ **What is the arrangement of collagen within a tendon and how does this contribute to the tendon's strength?**

Collagen lies in a parallel orientation and this gives the tendon great tensile strength.

○ **Describe the anatomy of a tendon from its most basic molecule to the tendon itself.**

Tropocollagen (composed of polypeptide chains) polymerize into bundles called collagen filaments. Filaments bundle to form a fibril. Fibrils bundle to form a primitive fiber which in turn bundles to form a fiber. These fibers bundle to form a fascicle. Fascicles are surrounded by an endotenon. These are gathered to form the tendon which is surrounded by the epitenon.

○ **To what degree does the tendon sheath contribute to tendon healing?**

Little if anything.

❍   **Are adhesions considered a complication of surgery after primary tendon repair? Explain.**

No. Adhesion formation is a normal process and an integral part of the healing process. However, they can become excessive and impede tendon function.

❍   **What are the two variables that Blix refers to on his contractile force curve?**

Tension versus length.

❍   **Muscles tend to produce their greatest force at what percentage of their resting length?**

120% of their resting length.

❍   **As muscle fibers shorten, what happens to tension on the Blix contractile force curve?**

Tension decreases.

❍   **When surgically approximating the ends of a severed tendon, what is the desired tension of the musculotendinous unit?**

Zero or physiological tension.

❍   **At what percentage of a muscle's resting length is zero tension present?**

Approximately 60% of their resting length.

❍   **How does the length of a lever arm affect force?**

A long lever arm will increase force – it allows for more torque to be produced.

❍   **What is the normal ratio of torque produced by the anterior and posterior leg muscles in controlling foot function?**

1:4 (anterior:posterior).

❍   **Regarding the above ratio, how is this discrepancy offset biomechanically?**

The anterior lever arm of the forefoot is long which increases the force of the anterior leg muscles compared to the short lever arm of the triceps through the posterior calcaneus.

❍   **What does the cross sectional mass of a tendon determine?**

Strength of the force.

❍   **When evaluating the relationship of joint axes to the various tendons, what does the proximity of a tendon to a joint axis determine?**

The proximity of a tendon to a joint axis will determine whether its force is primarily stabilizing or rotatory. The closer a tendon is to a joint axis, the more of a stabilizing force it will have. The further away it is, the more of a rotatory force it will have.

❍   **If the tendon synovial sheath is damaged or excised, can it repair itself or regenerate?**

Yes – excision of the sheath results in repair through the formation of granulation tissue (this tissue does not contribute to, nor interfere with, healing of tendon).

○   **In general, what are the ways that tendons can be attached in a tendon transfer?**

Tendon to tendon, tendon to periosteum, and tendon to bone.

○   **Describe the location of a skin incision in relation to a tendon when planning a tendon procedure? Why is it important to place the incision in this manner?**

The incision should not be directly over the tendon. When possible, it should be made parallel to local skin lines or relaxed skin tension lines. Incision planning in this manner is imperative to minimize the development of scar tissue which can interfere with free tendon movement.

○   **Describe the attachment of the transferred tendon fibers in the STATT procedure?**

The lateral fibers of the tibialis anterior are sutured to the peroneus tertius tendon (when present). If not present, the fibers can be attached to the cuboid bone laterally or into the fibers of the peroneus brevis tendon.

Range of motion. Range of motion is the key to rehabilitation since restoration of range of motion assists all other rehabilitation parameters, ie. strengthening, endurance, neuromuscular coordination, proprioception, skill training, etc.

○   **What are indicators for an athlete to return to activity?**

Full and pain-free range of motion.
Normal muscle strength vs. contralateral side.
Satisfactory muscular endurance.
Correction of muscle imbalances (strength ratios/flexibility).
Correction or rectification of pre-existing biomechanical flaws/faults.
Restoration of protective proprioception.
Completion of appropriate skill tests per particular sport/event.

TRAUMA

○ **At least how many views are necessary to confirm the diagnosis of a fracture?**

At least two.

○ **Are oblique views used to evaluate fracture fragment relationships?**

No – need functional views (angle and base of gait).

○ **Describe a spiral fracture?**

Fracture is spiral in relation to the longitudinal axis of the bone. The fracture line is usually at least 2 times longer than the transverse diameter of the bone in the central area of the fracture.

○ **What patient population does one usually see greenstick or torus fractures?**

Pediatric population – where the individual has not yet achieved full growth.

○ **Is there a difference between a stress fracture and pathologic fracture? Discuss.**

Pathologic fracture occurs in bone that has been weakened by a disease process. Stress fracture occurs in normal bone due to overuse or microtrauma.

○ **Describe a comminuted fracture.**

At least 3 fragments must be present for a fracture to be classified as comminuted. More than one fracture line exists in one bone.

○ **Does fracture location in cancellous versus cortical bone affect healing? Discuss.**

Yes. Cancellous has a better healing potential – has better osteogenic properties, large fracture surfaces, good soft tissue support, good vascularization and good inherent stability compared to cortical bone.

○ **Describe the circumstances needed for primary bone healing.**

Possible only with rigid internal fixation and excellent anatomical position.

○ **What type of healing would one see external bone callus formation, primary or secondary?**

Secondary.

○ **What relationships must one describe when describing a fracture?**

Length, location, angulation rotation, displacement, articular nature, stability, and direction fracture line.

○ **What is closed reduction?**

Manipulation of fracture fragments into normal alignment without the use of surgical incision.

❍   **Describe the mechanism performed for closed reduction.**

Increase the deformity, distract the fragments and reverse the deformity.

❍   **What is the purpose of increasing the deformity when performing closed reduction?**

Allows for soft tissue that is interposed between the fragments to be released.

❍   **Patient presents with a crush injury to the 2ⁿᵈ toe. A subungual hematoma is noted. X-ray reveals a transverse fracture of the distal phalanx. What is your next step in the treatment/evaluation of this patient?**

Nail bed must be examined for possibility of laceration. (Remove nail plate.)

❍   **The nail plate is removed in the above patient. A 0.5 cm laceration is noted upon inspection of the nail bed. How would this affect the classification and treatment of this patient?**

This is now considered an open fracture. Will need local wound care, tetanus prophylaxis and systemic antibiotic therapy.

❍   **Injuries involving nail bed tissue loss are categorized according to what as described by Rosenthal?**

Level of injury (Zones) and direction of tissue loss.

❍   **Describe the zones in the Rosenthal classification for nail bed tissue loss and distal digital tip injuries.**

Zone I is distal to distal phalanx, zone II is distal to lunula and zone III is proximal to the distal end of the lunula.

❍   **List the directions of nail bed tissue loss.**

Dorsal oblique, transverse, plantar oblique, axial and central/gouging.

❍   **Secondary intention healing would be a viable treatment option for which Rosenthal zone of injury?**

Zone I.

❍   **What are the two most common mechanisms of acute injury to the nail bed and its associated structures?**

Crushing injury and stubbing forces.

❍   **A patient presents s/p dropping a book on his great toe and as a subungual hematoma of 35 % of his nail. What is the recommended treatment for this?**

Remove the nail plate and inspect the nail bed for laceration. As a general rule, when greater than 25 to 35 % of the nail plate is involved, the above is recommended. Less than this can be treated by evacuation of the hematoma with a Bovie, hot paper clip or other means

❍   **Which sesamoid is most commonly fractured in the foot?**

Tibial sesamoid.

❍   **What are the radiographic features evaluated when differentiating a fractured sesamoid from a congenital partite sesamoid?**

The presence of irregular, jagged serrated lines of separation between fragments, the size of the injured sesamoid being similar to neighboring or corresponding contralateral sesamoids, fragments that are widely separated and/or abnormally positioned, longitudinally or obliquely oriented division lines between fragments, interruption or peripheral cortices and evidence of bone callus formation in follow-up radiographs.

❍   **Is healing usually a problem with a fractured sesamoid? Why?**

Yes because it is highly avascular. There is a high rate of non-unions with this fracture type.

❍   **What is the accepted mechanism of injury for a 1ˢᵗ MTPJ dislocation?**

Hyperextension force of the phalanx-sesamoid apparatus on the metatarsal.

❍   **Describe closed reduction for a dislocated 1ˢᵗ MTPJ.**

Distraction of toe, exaggerated dorsiflexion followed by forced plantarflexory relocation.

❍   **A patient presents with a dislocated 1ˢᵗ MPTJ. Radiographs reveal dorsal dislocation of the proximal phalanx and a normal sesamoid-to-sesamoid relationship with both sesamoids dorsal to the metatarsal. What type of reduction would most likely be required?**

Open reduction. The soft tissue around the joint maintains the position, and closed reduction is virtually impossible for this type of injury.

❍   **Which foot bones have the highest incidence for stress fractures?**

2ⁿᵈ metatarsal followed by the 3ʳᵈ metatarsal.

❍   **What is the most common fracture type of the 5ᵗʰ metatarsal?**

Avulsion type fracture involving the tuberosity of the 5ᵗʰ metatarsal (Stewart III).

❍   **Describe the location of the true Jones fracture?**

Located at the proximal diaphysis of the 5ᵗʰ metatarsal. It is supra articular.

❍   **The ligaments that attach the metatarsals to the tarsal bones are stronger plantarly or dorsally?**

Plantarly.

❍   **Describe Lisfranc's ligament?**

Interosseous ligament from medial cuneiform to 2ⁿᵈ metatarsal base.

❍   **Is the following statement true or false? There is no ligamentous attachment from the 1ˢᵗ to 2ⁿᵈ metatarsal base.**

This is true. All the other metatarsals are bound to one another by a series of transverse dorsal and plantar ligaments as well as intermetatarsal ligaments. The one exception is between the 1ˢᵗ and 2ⁿᵈ metatarsal bases.

❍   **What is a pathognomonic sign of Lisfranc dislocation?**

Diastasis between the 1st and 2nd metatarsal bases usually with a small avulsion fragment between the 1st and 2nd met bases.

❍   **If plain radiographs are unequivocal and you still suspect Lisfranc dislocation, what radiologic study would be indicated?**

Stress abduction views.

❍   **Describe the intrinsic stability of Lisfranc's joint.**

Tarsometatarsal joints form a bony arc from medial to lateral with extensive ligamentous support and the "keystone" nature of the 2nd metatarsal in which it is recessed at its base.

❍   **Discuss the Hardcastle classification system for Lisfranc injury.**

Classification system based on the injury pattern of metatarsal displacement. It is based on radiographic criteria and is useful in determining treatment necessary. Type A is total incongruity of the entire tarsometatarsal joint. This displacement can be in the sagittal (dorsoplantar) or transverse (lateral) planes or combined. Type B is partial incongruity. There are 2 types. B1 is medial displacement affecting the 1st metatarsal either alone or in combination of one or more of the 2nd, 3rd, or 4th metatarsals. B2 is lateral displacement of one or more of the four lesser metatarsals while the 1st is unaffected. Type C is divergent displacement involving partial or total incongruity of the joint. Type C has been also divided into 2 types signifying partial (C1) and total (C2) displacement.

❍   **What are the two mechanisms postulated for tarsometatarsal joint injury?**

Direct and indirect. Direct is crushing force on the dorsum of the foot. Indirect usually with forced forefoot plantarflexion and forefoot abduction of the foot. (Can be associated with forced forefoot dorsiflexion as well.)

❍   **What is the radiographic sign that is a pathognomonic indicator of nonunion?**

Sclerosis of the fracture ends.

❍   **What is the difference between a delayed union and a nonunion?**

The difference between these two is a factor of time. A Nonunion shows no progressive healing at a fracture site after 9 months s/p fracture while a delayed union is defined as a fracture site in which the healing has not advanced at the average rate for the location and type of fracture.

❍   **What are the two basic categories of nonunions seen radiographically?**

Atrophic (avascular) and Hypertrophic (vascular). Hypervascular also divided into elephant foot, horse foot and oligotrophic based on the amount of callus formation. Avascular divided into torsion wedge, comminuted, defect and atrophic.

❍   **An electric bone stimulator would most likely be beneficial for what type of nonunion as a primary form of treatment without surgical intervention.**

Hypertrophic (vascular).

❍   **How is an atrophic nonunion treated?**

Surgery to debride the fracture ends and a bone graft is inserted with fixation. A bone stimulator can also be applied along with cast immobilization.

○   **What is a pseudoarthrosis?**

A false joint formed at fracture site due to continued movement without proper immobilization.

○   **What are the four phases in the initial assessment of a trauma patient?**

Primary survey (Injuries that threaten life or limb are identified), Resuscitation (These life threatening injuries are treated), secondary survey (A systemic, in-depth evaluation of the patient from head to toe is performed with continuous reassessment of the patient's condition) and definitive care (Less serious injuries are managed).

○   **Discuss the primary survey when dealing with a trauma patient.**

ABC's: A = Airway maintenance is first step in trauma treatment. B = Breathing, C = Circulation with hemorrhage control (major concern is shock), D = Disability (assess neurologic status) and E = Exposure – completely undress patient and examine entire body.

○   **When maintaining an airway in a trauma patient, what must you assume until proved otherwise?**

Cervical spine injury until proved otherwise – do C-spine control.

○   **Patient presents with blistering wounds on the dorsum of her foot after spilling a cup of hot coffee on her foot. Classify this burn and describe the extent of the injury involved.**

These are 2nd degree burns. These are partial thickness affecting the epidermis and dermis but not penetrating through the basement membrane.

○   **Describe the recommended rewarming process that should be performed for a patient with frostbite.**

Rewarming should be done rapidly in water that is 38-44 degrees C (100 to 110 degrees F) for 15-20 minutes (up to 45 minutes if necessary). This is often painful and pain medications are often needed.

○   **What is the role of surgical debridement in frostbite injuries?**

It is difficult to assess the depth and extent of tissue injury so it is best to avoid early surgical debridement and instead allow the tissue to demarcate over several months. Amputations can then be performed. If infection and wet gangrene is present, however, early surgical intervention is necessary.

○   **What are the two types of epiphyses?**

Pressure epiphysis – located at ends of long bones and transmit pressure through the joint. They provide for longitudinal growth. Traction epiphysis or apophysis are sites of muscle/tendon attachment and are non-articular. These do not contribute to the longitudinal growth of bone.

○   **Describe the physis.**

This is a radiolucent cartilaginous plate located between the metaphysis and epiphysis in a long bone.

○   **What is the Thurston-Holland sign?**

This is also known as a "flag sign" and is seen in Salter Harris type II fractures in which a pattern with a triangular shaped metaphyseal fragment is created.

○   **Which Salter Harris injuries are considered intraarticular?**

Type III and Type IV.

O   **What is compression syndrome?**

Clinical entity resulting from elevated tissue pressure in a closed space confined by osseous and fascial structures. As the pressure increases, it compromises capillary blood perfusion that is needed for tissue viability. This leads to ischemia.

O   **What is the most common compartment in the leg involved in compartment syndrome?**

Anterior compartment followed by the deep posterior compartment.

O   **What is the degree of ischemia dependent on when dealing with compartment syndrome?**

Time.

O   **What are the six P's of compartment syndrome?**

Pain, pressure, paresthesia, paresis, pain with passive stretch, pulses present.

O   **At what pressure intracompartmental pressure would a fasciotomy be considered?**

Range of 30-45 mmHg with clinical symptoms.

O   **Describe the complication of myoglobulinuria in compartment syndrome.**

Occurs secondary to all the muscle necrosis. This can be fatal.

O   **Radiographically, how does one differentiate a fractured navicular tuberosity from a Type II accessory navicular?**

Accessory navicular is bilateral 90% of the time; the fracture is usually sharp with jagged edges while the accessory navicular has smooth rounded edges.

O   **Describe the usual mechanism of injury for a navicular tuberosity fracture.**

Usually an avulsion type fracture. When foot is forcibly everted, the posterior tibialis tendon exerts its force and causes the avulsion.

O   **What is Nutcracker syndrome?**

Severely displaced navicular tuberosity fracture caused by strong pronatory force will cause compression of calcaneo-cuboid joint producing occasional fracture of the cuboid and/or calcaneus.

O   **Describe the mechanism of injury for a dorsal avulsion fracture of the navicular.**

Plantarflexion with either inversion or eversion. With PF and eversion, the dorsal tibionavicular ligament (part of deltoid) avulses dorsal cortex of navicular bone at its insertion. With PF and inversion, the talonavicular ligament becomes stressed and avulses the dorsal cortex.

O   **Are dorsal lip (avulsion) fractures usually intra or extra-articular?**

Usually intraarticular because they contain articular cartilage.

❍   **Radiographically, there is an avulsion fracture at the medial aspect of the medial cuneiform. What is the most likely cause of this injury?**

Tibialis anterior.

❍   **What is the most commonly involved articular surface affected in calcaneal fractures?**

Posterior facet of calcaneus.

❍   **What structures are commonly impinged with lateral displacement of a calcaneus fracture.**

Peroneal tendons.

❍   **What is Mandor's sign?**

Hematoma and bruising that extend to the sole of the foot. This is common with calcaneal fractures and some consider it pathognomonic.

❍   **What angles must one measure when evaluating a calcaneal fracture?**

Bohler's angle and the crucial angle of Gissane.

❍   **What does an abnormal crucial angle of Gissane suggest?**

Abnormal relationship of the posterior facet to the anterior and middle facets is present.

❍   **What study would be best performed to determine the extent of an intraarticular calcaneal fracture?**

CT scan.

❍   **What radiographic view would be best to visualize a fracture of the anterior process of the calcaneus?**

Medial oblique view.

❍   **What structure most commonly causes the avulsion of the anterior process of the calcaneus?**

Bifurcate ligament.

❍   **What is the most common mechanism of injury for an anterior superior calcaneal fracture?**

Plantarflexion and inversion of the foot.

❍   **What are the two basic types of intraarticular calcaneal fractures?**

Tongue type and joint compression.

❍   **How are the above fractures differentiated?**

They are differentiated by the location of the secondary fracture line and by the shape of the fragments.

❍   **Describe the primary or vertical fracture line in an intraarticular calcaneal fracture.**

Superior to inferior extending from the vertex of Gissane's angle to the plantar aspect of the calcaneus. This is basically the same for both Tongue type and joint compression fractures.

O   If a patient has fallen from a height, what other injuries must be suspected besides a calcaneal fracture?

Lumbar spine, contralateral calcaneus, knees, hips, antebrachium and cranium. Also must suspect internal injury (lacerated spleen or kidney).

O   What mechanism of injury would most likely cause a medial talar osteochondral lesion?

Inversion of a plantarflexed foot.

O   Arthroscopy reveals a shallow, wafer shaped defect in the talar dome after injury. Where would this defect most likely be located on the talar dome and what was the most likely mechanism of injury?

Anterior or middle third of the talus in the lateral portion. Mechanism most likely was inversion of a dorsiflexed foot.

O   What is a shepherd's fracture?

Fracture of the posterolateral process of the talus. This is also sometimes called a Steida's fracture.

O   What is the most serious complication following a talar neck fracture?

Avascular necrosis.

O   What is Hawkins' sign?

Sign of viability of the blood supply following fracture/dislocation of the talus. There is subchondral bone atrophy due to hyperemia of the area of bone causing bone resorption.

O   What structure can be confused for a talar lateral tubercle fracture?

Os Trigonum.

O   Status post inversion ankle injury, radiographs reveal an avulsion fracture of the superolateral aspect of the calcaneus? What is the cause of this fracture?

Extensor digitorum brevis.

O   The anterior drawer sign evaluates the integrity of what structure?

Anterior talofibular ligament.

O   Arthrography of the ankle reveals dye passing superiorly through the syndesmosis. What does this suggest?

Definitive for diastasis.

O   Arthrography of the ankle reveals dye escaping to the lateral side of the lateral malleolus. What does this suggest?

Definitive for a tear of the lateral collateral ligaments.

○   **Mortise views of the ankle reveals increased soft tissue density over the lateral malleolus and a fracture lying parallel to the lateral malleolus. What is your diagnosis?**

Peroneal subluxation – Grade III.

○   **Describe the grades of peroneal subluxation.**

Grade I – the retinaculum and periosteum are separated from the fibrocartilaginous lip. Grade II – the fibrous lip was elevated along with the retinaculum. Grade III – a thin fragment of bone was elevated along with the fibrous lip.

○   **The Lauge-Hansen classification consists of two words. What do these words signify?**

First word (either supination or pronation) refers to position of the foot at the time of injury. The second word refers to the direction the talus moves in the ankle mortise.

○   **What is the Danis-Weber classification system based on?**

Anatomical position of the fibular fracture fragment in relation to the distal syndesmosis.

○   **Patient presents status post ankle injury. Radiographs reveal a transverse fracture of the fibula at the joint line and a vertical fracture of the medial malleolus. Classify this injury based on Lauge-Hansen.**

Supination-adduction injury Stage II.

○   **What is a Tillaux fracture?**

Avulsion of the tubercle of Tillaux-Chaput (anterolateral margin of the distal tibia).

○   **Avulsion of the distal fibula by the anterior inferior tibiofibular ligament is known as what?**

Wagstaffe fracture.

○   **Wagstaffe fracture would be seen in what stage of a supination eversion (external rotation) injury?**

Stage I.

○   **Radiographs reveal a spiral fracture of the fibula starting at the distal syndesmosis and a transverse fracture of medial malleolus. Classify this injury (Lauge Hansen)**

Supination-external rotation Stage IV.

○   **What is Volkmann's fracture?**

Avulsion fracture of the posterior malleolus.

○   **When should a Volkmann's fracture be fixated?**

If the fracture is 25% to 30% of the articular surface, fixate it.

○   **What is Vassal's principle as it applies to the ankle?**

When fibular fracture is reduced (correcting length and rotation) this should put the talus back into the mortise in perfect alignment. (This principle doesn't always perfectly reduce the medial malleolus and this usually needs further reduction.)

○   **What is a Maisonneuve fracture?**

This is a high fibular fracture seen in pronation-external rotation injuries.

○   **What stage injury is present if Maisonneuve fracture is noted?**

PER 3.

○   **A high fibular fracture is present with no other osseous injuries. What must be ruptured for this fracture to occur?**

Anterior tibiofibular ligaments, interosseous ligament, and deltoid ligament.

○   **Which lateral collateral ligaments are extra-capsular?**

Calcaneofibular.

○   **What is the function of inversion stress views?**

Done under anesthesia to determine the presence of an abnormal talar tilt (5 to 15 degrees is normal).

○   **What are some commonly missed fractures in ankle sprains?**

Base of the 5th metatarsal, anterior process of the calcaneus, Osteochondral dome fracture of talus, High fibular fracture, Posterior lateral distal tibia fracture (can be hidden by fibula), EDB avulsion fracture, and possibly a talar tubercle fracture.

○   **When is an open fracture considered contaminated verses infected?**

Open fractures are considered infected 8 hours post injury. They are considered contaminated up to this time.

○   **What are the two factors that determine the amount of kinetic energy that a projectile possesses (ie the amount of energy a bullet can deliver to tissue)?**

Mass and velocity. The formula $E=1/2mv^2$ determines the amount of energy possessed by a bullet.

○   **Discuss the Gustilo and Anderson classification.**

This is for open fractures and is based on the length of the wound and degree of associated soft tissue trauma. Type I is an open fracture with a wound less than one cm and usually a simple type fracture with minimal comminution. Type II has a wound greater than one cm without extensive soft tissue damage, flaps or avulsion and minimal comminution. Type III has extensive soft tissue damage including skin, muscle and neurovascular structures. Special considerations within Type III fractures include the following: Open segmental fracture irrespective of wound size, indicating a high-energy injury with more extensive soft tissue damage than is appreciated by the superficial wound, farm injuries, irrespective of wound size with soil contamination, high velocity gunshot wounds and close range shotgun wounds, fractures with neurovascular compromise, traumatic amputations, open fractures greater than 8 hours old.

○   **Why is the fact that a wound was due to a farm injury such an important consideration?**

This wound is Clostridial prone and can cause gas gangrene or tetanus.

O   **What is the antibiotic of choice for a type I, type II and type III Gustilo injury?**

For Gustilo type I and II injuries, a cephalosporin is the drug of choice. For a Type III wound, an aminoglycoside is added to the Cephalosporin to provide gram negative coverage.

MISCELLANEOUS

○ **List the common accessory bones seen in the foot.**

Os trigonum – posterior lateral process of the talus.
Os Peroneum – lateral inferior cuboid.
Os Tibiale Externum – medial inferior navicular tuberosity.
Os Vesalianum – base of 5th metatarsal, styloid area.
Os Navicularis – dorsal talonavicular joint.
Os calcaneus secondarium – anterior process of calcaneus.
Os sub sustentaculare – posterior to sustentaculum tali.

○ **List the components of an Operative Report.**

Date.
Patient Name, Patient Age.
Surgeon.
Assistant Surgeon.
Preoperative Diagnosis.
Postoperative Diagnosis.
Procedure.
Anesthesia.
Operation and Findings (Description of operation).
Signature.

○ **List the components of an Operative Note.**

S = Surgeon.
A = Assistant.
P = Pre-op diagnosis.
P = Post-op diagnosis.
P = Procedure.
A = Anesthesia.
H = Hemostasis.
E = Estimated blood loss.
M = Materials.
I = Injectables.
(P) = Pathology.
(C) = Complications.

○ **List the components of an Admit Note.**

Date.
Patient Name, Patient Age.
Admit to service of …
Diagnosis.
Condition.
Allergies.
Vital Signs.
Activities.
Nurses Orders.

Diet.
Ins/Outs.
Labs.
Medications.
Ancillary.
X-ray.

❍   **Describe how cabinets and x-ray viewing boxes are designed in the operating room.**

Recessed in the walls.

❍   **At what temperature is the operating room usually maintained?**

68 to 72 degrees F.

❍   **Describe the airflow (ventilation) system usually reserved for operating rooms where joint replacement with endoprostheses procedures are performed.**

Laminar flow unidirectional ventilation systems.

❍   **Describe what is contained in the sterile zone of an operating room facility.**

Actual operating room and sterile supply area.

❍   **The locker room facilities are located in which traffic zone of an OR facility?**

Protective area.

❍   **The scrub area is considered what traffic zone of an OR facility?**

Clean area.

❍   **What are the two methods for putting on sterile gloves?**

Open gloving and closed gloving.

❍   **What percentage of dextrose is in the IV replacement fluid D5W?**

5%.

❍   **What is the most common complication of IV therapy?**

Infiltration.

❍   **Crile, Kelly and Halstead are examples of what type of instrument.**

Hemostatic.

❍   **What is the function of the freer elevator?**

Reflection of periosteum off of bone.

❍   **At what is the relative humidity in the operating room maintained?**

50%.

BIBLIOGRAPHY

- Arndt, K: *Manual of Dermatologic Therapeutics with Essentials of Diagnosis*, 6th ed. Williams and Wilkins; 2002.
- Ashton R, Jones R, et al.: Juvenile plantar dermatosis. *Arch Derm* 121:225-228, 1985.
- Banks AS, et al.; *McGlamry's Comprehensive Textbook of Foot and Ankle Surgery*, 3rd ed. Williams and Wilkins; 2001.
- Bodman, M Miscellaneous Nail Presentations. In McCarthy, DJ (ed): Onychopathy. Clinics in Podiatric Medicine and Surgery, Philadelphia, W. B. Saunders Company, pages 327-346, April 1995.
- Bodman, M Pedal Nail and Skin Problems. In Robbins, JM (ed): Primary Podiatric Care Practice. Philadelphia, W.B. Saunders Company, 1994.
- Bono JV, Roger DJ, Jacobs RL: Surgical Arthrodesis of neuropathic feet: A Salvage procedure. Clin Orthop 296, 14, 1993.
- Caputo GM, Joshi N, Weitekamp MR: Foot infections in patients with diabetes. *Am Fam Physician* 56(1): 195-202, 1997.
- Clohisy DR, Thompson RC: Fractures associated with neuropathic arthropathy in adults who have juvenile-onset diabetes. *J Bone Joint Surg* 70 1192, 1988.
- Dahlin's Bone Tumors, General Aspects in Data on 11,087 Cases, 5th ed. , Krishnan Unni, Lippincott-Raven Publishers, Philadelphia, NY, 1996.
- Dawber, RPR, Baran, R: *Diseases of the Nails and Their Management*, Boston, Blackwells Scientific Publications; 1984.
- De Valentine S, *Foot and Ankle Disorders in Children*, Churchill Livingstone Inc.; 1992.
- DeFeo WT, Jay RM: Osteomyelitis associated with peripheral vascular disease secondary to diabetes mellitus. *JFoot Surg* 15(4):159-65, 1976.
- Devillers A, Moisan A, Hennion F, Garin E, Poitier JY, Bourguet P: Contribution of technetium-99m hexamethylpropylene amine oxime labeled leukocyte scintigraphy to the diagnosis of diabetic foot infection. *Eur J Nucl Med* 25(2): 132-8, 1998.
- *Dorland's Illustrated Medical Dictionary*, W. B. Saunders Co., Philadelphia, PA, 1974.
- Eckman MH, Greenfield S, Mackey WC, Wong JB, Kaplan S, Sullivan L, Dukes K, Pauker SG: Foot infections in diabetic patients. Decision and cost-effectiveness analyses. *JAMA* 273(9): 712-20,1995.
- Edelman D, Hough DM, Glazebrook KN, Oddone EZ: Prognostic value of the clinical examination of the diabetic foot ulcer. *J Gen Intern Med* 12(9): 537-43, 1997.
- Edmonds ME: *A Practical Manual of Diabetic Foot Care*, Blackwell Publishers; 2004.
- Fitzpatrick, JE, Aeling JL. Aeling: *Dermatology Secrets*, Hanley &Belfus, Inc.; 1996.
- Fitzpatrick, TB: *Atlas of Dermatology in General Medicine*, McGraw-Hill Co.; 1996.
- Garcia-Diaz JB, Pankey GA: *Contemporary Diagnosis and Management of Diabetic Foot Infections*, Handbooks in Healthcare Company; 2001.
- Gerbert J: *Textbook of Bunion Surgery*, 2nd ed., W.B. Sanders; 2000.
- Giurini JM, Applications and use of in-shoe orthoses in the conservative management of Charcot foot deformity. *Clin Podiatr Med* 11(2): 27 I, 1994.
- Grayson ML, Gibbons GW, Balogh K, Levin E, Karchmer AW: Probing to bone in infected pedal ulcers. A clinical sign of underlying osteomyelitis in diabetic patients. *JAMA* 273(9): 721-3, 1995.
- Guhl JF, et al.: *Foot and Ankle Arthroscopy*, 3rd ed. Springer Verlag; 2003.
- Gumann G: *Fractures of the Foot and Ankle*, W.B. Sanders; 2004.
- Hetherington V: *Hallux Valgus and Forefoot Surgery*, Churchill Livingstone; 1994.
- Klippel JH ed.: *Primer On The Rheumatic Diseases*, 12th ed. Arthritis Foundation; 2001.
- Kitaoka HB, Ravin D: *Master Techniques in Orthopaedic Surgery: The Foot and Ankle*, Williams and Wilkens; 2002.
- Kozak GP, Campbell DR, Frykberg RG; *Management of Diabetic Foot Problems*, 2nd ed., W.B. Sanders; 1995.
- Kumagi SG, Mahoney CR, Fitgibbons TC, McMullen ST, Connolly TL, Henkel L: Treatment of diabetic neuropathic foot ulcers with two-stage debridement and closure. *Foot Ankle Intl* 9(3):160-5, 1998.

- Larcos G, Brown ML, Sutton RT: Diagnosis of osteomyelitis of the foot in diabetic patients: value of 111 In-leukocyte scintigraphy. *Am JRoentgenol* 157(3): 527-31, 1991.
- Lavery LA, Harkless LB, Ashry HR, Feider-Johnson K: Infected puncture wounds in adults with diabetes: risk factors for osteomyelitis. *J Foot Ankle Surg* 33(6):561-6,1994.
- Lavery LA, Sariaya M, Ashry H, Harkless LB: Microbiology of osteomyelitis in diabetic foot infections. *J Foot Ankle Surg* 34(1):61-4, 1995.
- Lee MS, Hofbauer MH: Evaluation and Management of Lateral Ankle Injuries. Clinics in Podiatric Medicine and Surgery 16(4): 659, 1999.
- Lesko P, Maurer RC: Talonavicular dislocations and midfoot arthropathy in neuropathic diabetic feet: natural course and principles of treatment. *Clin Orthop* 240: 226,1989.
- Levesque J: *A Clinical Guide to Primary Bone Tumors*, 1st ed, Williams and Wilkins; 1998.
- Lorimer DL, French G: *Neale's Disorders of the Foot: Diagnosis and Management*, 6th ed. W.B. Sanders; 2002.
- Lipsky B Osteomyelitis of the foot in diabetic patients. *Clin Infect Dis* 25(6): 1318-26, 1997.
- Mandy A: *Psychosocial Approaches to Podiatry*. Churchill Livingston; 2003.
- Marcinko DE: *Osteomyelitis in Comprehensive Textbook of Foot Surgery*. 2nd ed., Williams and Wilkins; 1992.
- Marcus CD, Ladam-Marcus VJ, Leone J, Maigrange D, Bonnet-Gausserand FM, Menanteau BP: MR imaging of osteomyelitis and neuropathic osteoarthropathy in the feet of diabetics. *Radiographics* 16(6):1337-48, 1996.
- McCluskey LF, Webb LB: Compression and Entrapment Neuropathies of the Lower Extremity, Clinics in Podiatric Medicine and Surgery, Vol. 16 No. 1, January 1999.
- McGlamry D: *Comprehensive Textbook of Foot Surgery,* 2nd ed., Williams and Wilkins; 1992.
- Morgan JM, Biehl WC, Wagner FW: Management of neuropathic neuropathy with the Charcot restraint orthotic walker. *Clin Orthop* 296: 58,1993.
- Morrison WB, Schweitzer ME, Batte WG, Radack DP, Russel KM: Osteomyelitis of the foot: relative importance of primary and secondary MR imaging signs. *Radiology* 207(3):625-32, 1998.
- Murphy GP, et. al: *Clinical Oncology*, 2nd ed.,The American Cancer Society, 1995.
- Myerson M: *Foot and Ankle Disorders,* W.B. Sanders Co.; 1998.
- Oyen WJ, Netten PM, Letomens JA, Claessens RA, Lutterman JA, van der Vliet JA, Goris RJ, van der Meer JW, Corstens FH: Evaluation of infectious diabetic foot complications with indium-111-labeled human nonspecific immunoglobulin G. *J Nucl Med* 33(7):1330-6, 1992.
- Papa J, Myerson M, Girard P: Salvage, with arthrodesis, in intractable diabetic neuropathic arthropathy of the foot and ankle. *J Bone Joint Surg* 75A(I 2): 1056, 1993.
- Pittet D, Wyssa B, Herter-Clavel C, Kursteiner K, Vaucher J, Lew PD: Outcome of diabetic foot infections treated conservatively: a retrospective cohort study with long-term follow-up. *Arch Intern Med* 159(8): 851-6, 1999.
- Rooks MD: Coverage problems of the foot and ankle. *Orthop Clin North Am* 20(4): 723-36, 1989.
- Sanders L J, Frykberg RG: "Diabetic Neuropathic Osteoarthropathy: Charcot Foot," in the High Risk Foot in Diabetes Mellitus, ed. by ME Levin, LW O'Neal, JH Bowker, 5th ED, Churchill Livingstone, New York, 1991.
- Scurran BL, ed., *Foot and Ankle Trauma*, Churchill Livingstone;1989.
- Staheli L: *Pediatric Orthopaedic Secrets*, 2nd ed., Hanley & Belfus, Inc.; 2002.
- Steck WD: Wet foot dry foot syndrome. *Cleveland Clinic Quarterly*, Summer, p145-149, 1983.
- Thordarson DB: *Foot and Ankle (Orthopaedic Surgery Essentials)*, Williams and Wilkins; 2004.
- Venkatesan P, Lawn S, Macfarlane RM, Fletcher EM, Finch RG, Jeffcoate WJ: Conservative management of osteomyelitis in the feet of diabetic patients. *Diabet Med* 14(6): 487-90, 1997.
- Weatherford ML: *Podiatry Sourcebook*, Omnigraphics, 2001.